A Self-Instructional Guide:

SURGICAL COMPLICATIONS

by

Dale S. Bloomquist, DDS, MSD
James R. Hooley, DDS
Robert J. Whitacre, MS, DDS

A Self-Instructional Guide:
SURGICAL COMPLICATIONS
Third Edition
(ISBN #0-89939-041-2)

AUTHORS

DALE S. BLOOMQUIST, DDS, MSD, Department of Oral and Maxillofacial Surgery, School of Dentistry, University of Washington, Seattle, Washington.

JAMES R. HOOLEY, DDS, Dean and Professor of Oral and Maxillofacial Surgery, School of Dentistry, University of California at Los Angeles, Los Angeles, California.

ROBERT J. WHITACRE, MS, DDS, Educational Consultant, Department of Oral and Maxillofacial Surgery, School of Dentistry, University of Washington, Seattle, Washington.

This book is one of a series of self-instructional textbooks designed to teach concepts of oral surgery and related disciplines to dental students, dental practitioners and dental auxiliaries. The series title of **A Self-Instructional Guide to Oral Surgery in General Dentistry** was formerly used to describe this series; however, the title has been altered to reflect the fact that the series has grown to include additional specialties. This book series includes the following self-instructional book titles:

1. **Instruments Used for Oral Surgery**
2. **The Removal of Teeth**
3. **Medications Used in Oral Surgery**
4. **Surgical Complications**
5. **Dental Asepsis**
6. **Assessment of and Surgery for Impacted Third Molars**
7. **Pre-Prosthetic Surgery**
8. **Principles of Biopsy**
9. **Diagnosis and Treatment of Odontogenic Infections**

published by

Stoma Press, Inc.

13231 42nd Avenue NE
Seattle, WA 98125
(206) 365-2665

Typeset By

CASTEEL TYPESETTING
18316 1st NE
Seattle, WA 98155
(206) 363-9054

Printed By

ATOMIC PRESS
1421 N 34th
Seattle, WA
(206) 632-0550

EDITORIAL CONSULTANTS

MESSAGE TO LEARNER

When reading a standard textbook, it is often difficult for you to know exactly what the important content is. It is difficult to separate areas that are essential for you to understand from those that are nice to know. You may often have thought you knew the material but could not apply it when presented with the clinical situation. You may also have had a problem during examinations when instructors asked you questions that were **not** covered in your reading.

In writing this book, considerable time and effort have been invested in creating a feedback system for you to monitor your learning progress. We have included a section termed "overview and objectives" which states the essential kinds of performances or knowledge you can expect to gain from reading the contents and completing the study exercises. We have included a **"Pre-Test"** for each unit. The "Pre-Test" is intended to show you what you don't know about the content of the unit. It is difficult for you to see learning take place unless you have both a "before" and "after" demonstration. You should retake the pre-tests following completion of each unit.

The **study exercises** are designed for different levels of learning. The **first level** of study exercises are of the "fill in the blank" type. The blanks usually include "key" words or phrases taken from the content preceding the study exercise.

The **second level** of study exercises is designed as problem-solving tasks. Generally these take a small piece of a larger concept and allow you to focus your attention on mastery of the piece. Learning one piece at a time is similar to learning your multiplication tables. The small pieces are then assimilated into larger concepts which you can learn with ease.

The **third level** of questions are simulations of clinical problems that you will be faced with in treating patients. Having completed the previous study exercises, you should be able to adequately cope with these. These are the most important study exercises because they resemble the real world of dentistry. Through adequate analysis and planning, complications or surprises during surgery can be greatly reduced. These are similar to "story problems" in mathematics.

The study exercises are **extremely important** and you should take the time to **write the answers** in the blanks or spaces provided. You may be tempted to mentally answer the questions or skip them entirely to save time. You will **retain more of the information** you have read with much **less effort** if you take the time to write out the answers as you proceed. Considerable research in self-instructional design and learning has shown the importance of answering such study questions.

Although we have had considerable input from many people in writing this book, we by no means imply that these techniques, instruments or concepts are the "only way." Your oral surgeon or instructors may wish to deviate from the methods described, especially with regard to specific clinical situations.

TABLE OF CONTENTS

OVERVIEW AND OBJECTIVES

UNIT I

This unit discusses the four most common types of soft-tissue injuries that can occur during oral-surgical procedures, their causes, and treatment.

After completing this unit, you will:

1. State the four common types of soft-tissue injuries that can occur while performing intra-oral surgical procedures.

2. Describe procedures for reducing the risk of each of the above soft-tissue injuries.

3. Describe procedures for treating each of the types of soft tissue injuries.

UNIT II

Accidental injuries due to uncontrolled force or improper placement of instruments may occur during the removal of teeth. This unit deals with the most common types of these injuries in terms of cause, prevention, and treatment.

After completing this unit you will:

1. Describe the method discussed for reducing the risk for fracturing the maxillary alveolus during tooth extraction.

2. Describe the method of treatment for the following situations if they should occur during the routine extraction of teeth:
    a. Bone removed with the tooth with no soft tissue attached.
    b. Fractured alveolus that has bone still attached to periosteum.
    c. Larger fracture of the maxillary tuberosity with periosteum still attached.
    d. Inadvertent fracture of the mandible.

3. Name three possible injuries to adjacent teeth that can occur during extraction procedures as discussed in this unit.

4. For each of the five injuries named above, describe methods of prevention and treatment, according to this unit.

5. Describe methods to prevent root fracture and displaced teeth or roots during extractions.

6. Describe treatment for a displaced tooth or root.

UNIT III

This unit deals with complications affecting the maxillary sinus, temporomandibular joint, and injuries caused by broken instruments.

After completing this unit, you will describe:

1. The preferred method to determine the presence of an oro-antral communication following a maxillary extraction.

2. Treatment for an oro-antral opening.

3. Treatment for an oro-antral fistula.

4. The procedures designed to reduce trauma to the temporomandibular joint during routine extraction of teeth.

5. Treatment for a patient complaining of pain elicited from the temporomandibular joint following a routine extraction.

6. Treatment for the dislocation of the condyle from the glenoid fossa in terms of:

   a. Dentist position relative to the patient.
   b. Thumb and finger placement.
   c. Direction of rotation of the mandible.

7. Methods of prevention and treatment for broken needles.

8. Methods of prevention and treatment for broken elevator tips.

UNIT IV

This unit discusses post-operative management of patients.

After completing this unit, you will:

1. Describe how to present information to the patient regarding post-operative self-care

2. Describe what to explain to your patient for the post-operative management of:

   a. Bleeding
   b. Swelling
   c. Discomfort
   d. Diet
   e. Medication
   f. Oral hygiene
   g. Sleeping and physical activity

UNIT V

Most post-operative complications can be attributed to poor pre-operative planning or mishandling of the patient during surgery. This unit discusses pre-operative procedures that can minimize post-operative hemorrhage problems, methods of controlling such hermorrhage, treatment of fibrinolytic alveolitis (dry socket), what to do if you inadvertently injure a major nerve, and how to handle surgical wound dehiscence problems.

After completing this unit you will:

1. Tell why each of the following seven questions you should ask your patient will help alert you to a potential bleeding disorder.

    a. Have you had any period of prolonged bleeding?

    b. Have you had liver disease?

    c. Do you have hypertension (high blood pressure)?

    d. Are you presently on any anticoagulant therapy?

    e. Do you bruise easily?

    f. Do you have anemia?

    g. Has anyone in your family had a history of bleeding problems?

2. List two rules in planning surgery that can help you prevent post-operative bleeding problems.

3. State two precautions you should take during surgery to reduce post-operative bleeding.

4. List four laboratory tests that should be used to help rule out bleeding problems and describe the significance of each.

5. Describe two things that can be done to decrease the possibility that a post-surgical bleeding problem will develop once your patient has left your office.

6. List three things you should evaluate if a patient returns with a complaint of post-operative hemorrhage.

7. List three methods of controlling bone bleeding.

8. List three methods of controlling soft-tissue bleeding.

9. List three clinical signs and symptoms of fibrinolytic alveolitis.

10. List five suggestions, according to this unit, that can be followed to decrease the incidence of fibrinolytic alveolitis.

11. Explain how fibrinolytic alveolitis should be treated.

12. State what treatment is necessary if bone spicules are not removed during surgery and are causing your patient discomfort.

13. State how to avoid injury to the inferior alveolar, lingual, and mental nerves during surgery.

14. State which of the following nerves may pose problems to the patient if injured during surgery.
    a. long buccal

    b. inferior alveolar

    c. lingual

    d. nasopalatine

    e. mental

UNIT I

SOFT TISSUE INJURIES

Introduction
Mucosal tears
Punctures
Inadvertent incisions
Heat injuries
Abrasion & avulsion injuries
Crush injuries

PRE-TEST FOR UNIT I

- *Answer the following questions.*
- *Check your answers against those on Page 10.*
  If all are correct, proceed to Unit II.
  If you got some answers wrong, turn to Page 10 and begin Unit I.

Questions:

1. *The inadvertent tearing of soft tissue while utilizing a flap procedure is usually due to* _______________

2. *Treatment of a mucosal tear consists of* _______________
____

3. *What is the treatment for a puncture wound accidentally made in the soft palate with a 301 dental elevator?* _______________
____

4. *While using a #15 Bard Parker blade during a surgical procedure you accidentally made a 3 mm incision in the upper lip. How would you treat this injury?* _______________
____

5. *What precautions should be taken when handling instruments fresh out of the autoclave while wearing surgical gloves?* _______________
____

6. *Following the utilization of a Turbo-Jet handpiece, you note that a portion of the lower lip has been abraded away. What is the proper treatment?* _______________
____

7. *A patient calls your office the day after you extracted #17 using forceps, complaining of a large bruise on her lower lip. How might this injury have occurred?* _______________
____

CONTENTS FOR UNIT I

SOFT TISSUE INJURIES

INTRODUCTION

Six primary types of injuries that can occur to the soft tissue during intraoral surgical procedures are:

- **Mucosal tears**
- **Punctures**
- **Inadvertent scalpel incisions**
- **Heat injuries**
- **Abrasion and avulsion injuries**
- **Crush injuries**

MUCOSAL TEARS

One of the most common reasons for inadvertent soft tissue tears in the oral cavity during surgery is careless retraction of a flap. Usually this is due to a surgeon's attempt to work in an area with inadequate access. Adequate exposure, therefore, is one of the primary methods by which this type of injury can be prevented.

Uncontrolled pressure applied to a periosteal elevator is also a common reason for a soft tissue tear. Lacerations of the soft tissue can be prevented when elevating a full thickness flap by a careful prying action of the periosteal elevator.

Treatment

Treatment consists of carefully closing the wound with sutures. If you have the unfortunate occasion to tear the flap so that the blood supply is compromised, the proper treatment is to replace the flap to achieve primary closure and secure in place with sutures. Fortunately, because of the good vascularity of the face and oral cavity, most of these flaps will survive.

PUNCTURES

Uncontrolled force may result in puncture injury to soft tissue. This usually occurs when a sharp instrument such as a 301 elevator slips off the tooth and penetrates the soft tissues. Usually the force is directed toward the palatal tissues in the maxilla and toward the lingual in the mandible. The force is usually directed posteriorly so, when slipping occurs, the posterior palatal tissues or the lateral pharyngeal wall are the sites most frequently involved.

Prevention

Prevention involves careful control of forces when using these types of instruments.

Treatment

Treatment includes irrigation of the wound and close follow-up of the patient until the area heals. There is usually no need to suture the wound. Suturing the puncture may block drainage from the depth of the wound. Leaving the wound open will allow drainage to occur, and the area will heal by secondary intention.

INADVERTENT INCISIONS

Occasionally, usually through lack of attention, you may accidentally nick or incise tissues of the lips or cheeks.

Prevention

When using a scalpel in the oral cavity, it is imperative that you be constantly alert to the location of the sharp edge of the blade from the time you pick it up until you return it to the tray. The lips are the most frequent site of inadvertent incisions.

Treatment

Usually such incisions are very small and do not require suturing. If, however, the incision is deep, it should be sutured, and the usual principles of wound management followed.

HEAT INJURIES

Heat injuries are usually due to the use of instruments "hot out of the autoclave." An instrument that feels warm through your rubber glove is usually hot enough to cause soft tissue damage.

Prevention

Allow instruments to cool prior to use. If you must use a recently sterilized "hot" instrument during surgery, you can speed cooling by immersing in cool sterile saline.

Management

No treatment is currently available. You may find it helpful to apply vaseline. If scarring results after initial healing, you may wish to refer the patient to a specialist for scar revision.

ABRASION AND AVULSION INJURIES

The lips and cheeks can be injured by rotating long-shanked burs. The rotating shafts may abrade the epithelieum from the mucosa. Occasionally, avulsive wounds (tearing out a segment of tissue) of the lip can result from the use of rotary instruments.

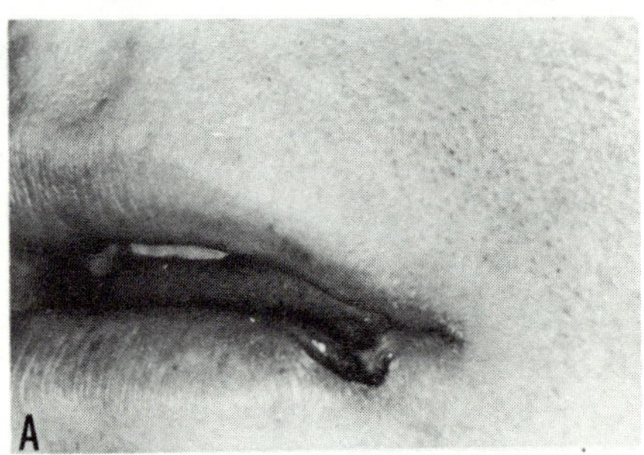

Figure 1. A. Avulsion of vermilion border of lower lip. The avulsion was caused by the rotating shank of a turbo-jet handpiece.

Prevention

You can prevent these injuries by retracting the lip whenever you use rotary instruments (e.g., when sectioning teeth or removing bone). You should also be aware at all times of the location of your burs in relation to soft tissues.

Treatment

Little can be done for abrasion and avulsion injuries other than palliative treatment and the usual follow-up care. Rarely, an avulsive injury of the lip will require secondary revision.

CRUSH INJURIES

During extraction procedures patients will frequently show great alarm and complain of pain in an area remote from the area of surgery. If they are able to speak they may say "you are pinching my lower lip." Impinging on the lower lip with forceps while extracting maxillary posterior teeth is a common problem and if your patient is not anesthetized in this region he will usually complain before significant crush damage is inflicted. On the other hand, if the lower lip is anesthetized, the forceps may inflict serious crush injury before you or your patient become aware of the problem.

Treatment

There is usually no treatment necessary other than palliative. This injury can be very annoying to your patients and they will no doubt wonder if you were somewhat careless during surgery.

When a surgeon attempts to work in an area to which there is inadequate access, he/she is likely to cause a_______________________in the mucosa. Applying (controlled/uncontrolled) ____________________force to a periosteal elevator may also cause a _______________________ in the mucosa. Two methods for minimizing the risk for mucosal tears are:

1. *Reflecting a full thickness mucoperiosteal flap that allows for adequate__________ ____________________to the surgical procedure.*

2. *When reflecting full thickness flaps with a periosteal elevator, use a ____________ action with care.*

Generally speaking, the procedure for treating a mucosal tear is to ____________________ the flap with sutures.

Punctures are usually caused by uncontrolled____________________using elevators. Often the structure damaged is the_______________________________________wall following the slippage of an elevator during luxation of a tooth. This may be prevented by controlling all ____when using elevators.

Following an accidental puncture you (should/should not)____________________________suture the wound. Closing the puncture may______________________________any natural drainage that may develop from the deposition of bacteria into the deeper tissues. Close patient ____________________is necessary to detect complications should they arise.

Inadvertent incisions in the oral cavity, face, etc. may result from ___________________ of scalpel blades. Most often these are____________________and need not be closed with sutures. Larger wounds, however, require closure with the appropriate________________ material.

Heat injuries to lips and mucosa are usually caused by ______________________________.

Heat injuries are managed primarily by applying_____________________________because no treatment is currently available. If scarring occurs, you may wish to _________________ ____________________________________.

Abrasion and avulsion injuries can result from____________________________. Treatment for these injuries includes____________________care and__________________________.

You should be constantly aware of the danger of inflicting crush injuries. An area where this injury is common is____. This can be a serious problem if your patient has received ___________________________ of the mandible because ____.

Now re-take the Pre-test, Unit I, and progress as indicated.

UNIT II

DAMAGE TO BONE AND TEETH

Introduction
Fracture of Maxillary Alveolus
    Examination of pre-operative
      radiographs
    Use of controlled force
    Supporting the alveolus
    Removal of buccal bone and
      sectioning of teeth
    Fracture of maxillary tuberosity
Fracture of the mandible

Injuries to adjacent teeth
    Partial avulsion of the adjacent
      tooth
    Fracture of cusps, incisal edges
      or restoration
    Extraction of the wrong tooth
Complications associated with
    individual tooth removal
    Fractured roots
    Displaced teeth
    Displaced molar roots

PRE-TEST FOR UNIT II

- *Cover the answers on page 16.*
- *Answer the following questions.*
- *Check your answers against those on page 16.*

    If all are correct, proceed to Unit III.
    If you got some answers wrong, turn to Page 16 and begin Unit II.

Questions:

1. *List three steps that should be taken to decrease the possiblity of fracturing the alveolus.*
    a. ____
    b. ____
    c. ____

2. *During the extraction of a second maxillary molar, you note that a large section of the alveolus was removed with the apex of the tooth. Also, you notice that a portion of this piece of bone is a smooth, partially concave surface about 6 mm long. How should the patient be treated?*

    ____

    ____

3. *While removing a maxillary first molar, you detect that a large portion of the maxillary alveolus has been fractured during luxation of the tooth.*
    a. How would you proceed with the extraction? ___________________________
    b. How would you manage the fractured alveolus? ___________________________

4. *During the removal of an erupted maxillary third molar you note that a whole fragment of alveolus including the second molar suddenly moves with the forceps. The mucosa is still attached to the bone. What is your treatment?*

5. *While using a 34 elevator to remove the mesial half of a horizontally impacted third molar, you hear a sudden crack and observe a fracture line running down the lingual cortical plate. Putting pressure on the mandible or having the patient bite causes this fracture line to expand. What is your diagnosis and treatment?*

6. *While removing the second mandibular premolar on a 12 year-old child with an elevator, you notice that the first premolar has suddenly been partially evulsed. What is the treatment?*

7. *While removing a mesioangular impaction, you accidentally fracture the distal half of a large amalgam of the second molar.*
   a. What is the treatment?
   b. What should you have done prior to beginning the procedure?

8. *You have been asked to remove the right maxillary second premolar for orthodontic therapy on a 12-year-old child. During the procedure you become aware that you accidentally extracted the right maxillary first premolar. How should you handle the situation?*

9. *When examining radiographs of a tooth prior to extraction, what conditions indicate increased danger for root fracture?*
   a.　　　　　　　　　　*d.*
   b.　　　　　　　　　　*e.*
   c.　　　　　　　　　　*f.*

10. *What complication can occur when trying to remove an impacted maxillary third molar that has a conically shaped root?*

11. *You have just attempted to split a mandibular third molar with a chisel and mallet. However, instead of splitting, the tooth suddenly disappeared inferiorly. What has happened and how should it be treated?*

PRE-TEST — UNIT II, Answers

1. a. Examine pre-operative x-rays
    b. Control force during extraction
    c. Support the alveolus during extraction
2. Care should be taken to primarily close the soft tissue over the extraction site, since this is the description of an avulsed alveolus that includes a portion of the sinus floor.
3. a. Lay a small flap that does not devitalize the bone fragment and section the tooth allowing removal in separate pieces.
    b. Using your maxillary pinch grasp, squeeze the fractured alveolus into place and allow time for it to repair.
4. Stabilize the segment and the teeth with an acrylic or wire splint for about six weeks.
5. If you know how to treat fractured mandibles, this should be treated in a routine manner with an Eric arch bar. However, if you are unfamiliar with the procedure, your patient should be referred to an oral surgeon for treatment.
6. The tooth should be stabilized with either wire or wire and acrylic.
7. a. After finishing the surgical procedure, temporary restorative material should be placed and then replaced with a more permanent material after the surgical site heals.
    b. Before surgery, advise patient of possible fracture of the restoration during surgery.
8. Contact the orthodontist and explain what has happened. He may be able to alter his treatment without difficulty. If not, replace the tooth and stabilize it with wire and acrylic and advise the patient and his parent(s) of what has occurred.
9. a. Slender roots   d. Ankylosed roots
    b. Curved roots   e. Devitalized teeth
    c. Divergent roots   f. Dense alveolar bone
10. Displacing the tooth either into the sinus or into the infratemporal fossa.
11. The tooth has been displaced into the submandibular space and the patient should be referred to an oral surgeon as soon as possible for removal.

CONTENTS FOR UNIT II

DAMAGE TO BONE AND TEETH

INTRODUCTION
Damage to teeth or investing bone is usually due to the use of uncontrolled force or improper placement of instruments. Often you can reduce the probability of hard tissue damage through careful pre-operative case analysis and subsequent modification of your usual surgical technique.

FRACTURE OF THE MAXILLARY ALVEOLUS
The inadvertent removal of bone with an extraction of a tooth occurs with significant frequency in routine exodontia.

Prevention
Much of this bone loss, however, can be prevented by:
- Examination of pre-operative radiographs.
- Use of controlled force during the extraction procedure.
- Supporting the alveolus during the extraction.
- Removal of buccal bone and sectioning of teeth.

Examination of Pre-operative Radiographs
The principal areas of concern are the maxillary sinus and the tuberosity. Specific problems related to these regions are described elsewhere in this chapter.

Use of Controlled Force
Using excessive force in an extraction procedure can result in either fracturing of the tooth root or fracturing of the supporting alveolar bone. You should always take care to carefully luxate the tooth initially to allow expansion of a socket, especially in the maxilla, before exerting the force necessary for removing the tooth. Determining how much force should be applied comes largely through clinical experience.

Supporting the Alveolus
Since many of the fractures occur in the maxilla, it is wise to grasp the alveolus around the tooth while forces are being applied with either elevator or forceps. With the fingers in this pinch grasp position, as described in the chapter, "The Removal of Teeth," it is possible both to support the alveolus and feel any abnormal movement of the bone which may precede a fracture. With fingers positioned this way, you will be aware of a fracture, and can take steps to repair the damage.

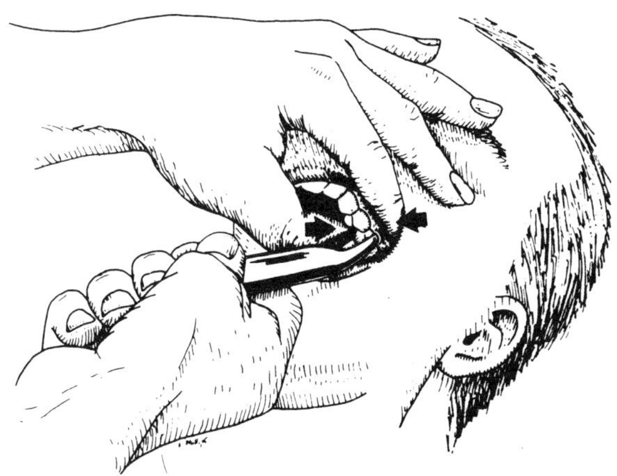

Figure 2. Maxillary Pinch Grasp

Removal of Buccal Bone and Sectioning of Teeth
The following illustrations will serve as a reminder that it is often necessary to remove buccal bone and section teeth in order to prevent a fracture of the alveolar bone or the tooth.

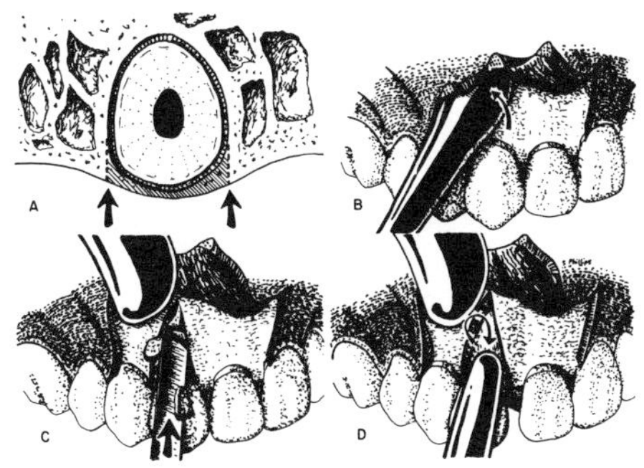

Figure 3. Surgical extraction of a maxillary canine. A. Note the relatively thin labial bone covering the convexity of the tooth and the thick bone at the mesiolabial and distolabial aspects of the roots. B. A mucoperiosteal flap is reflected. C. Labial bone is removed with a monobevel chisel. D. The tooth is extracted with a forceps.

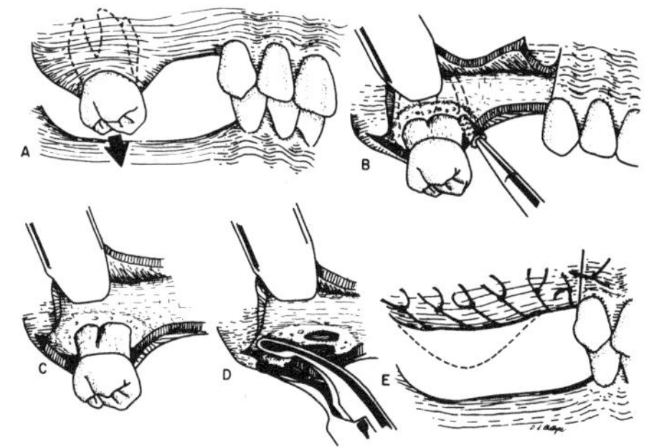

Figure 4. Prevention of tuberosity fracture caused by the extraction of an overerupted isolated molar. A. Overerupted isolated molar. B. and C. Flap reflected and buccal bone removed to prevent fracture. D. Excessive bone is removed with rongeurs. E. The soft tissues are trimmed and sutured.

Treatment
Bone that has been completely removed from soft tissue
When bone is completely removed with a tooth it usually cannot be replaced. Treatment consists of carefully repositioning the soft tissue flap to cover as much of the exposed surface as possible. If there is a jagged edge left by the fractured bone, it is wise to smooth it with a rongeurs or bone file prior to the soft tissue closure. If the removed bone is at the apex of the tooth and appears to contain a portion of the sinus floor, care should be taken to primarily close the soft tissue over the extraction site. In any event, **DO NOT PROBE** the socket.

Bone Still Attached to Periosteum
A fracture discovered before bone is removed from the soft tissue should be handled by separating the bone from the tooth without displacing the periosteum and its blood supply. This may require either careful elevation of the bone away from the tooth, or sectioning the tooth with a bur. It does not, however, require laying a flap over the fracture. This will devitalize the bone fragment and compromise its chances for survival. With the tooth removed from the socket, bone fragments can be positioned and supported by sutures.

Fracture of Maxillary Tuberosity
Fracture of the tuberosity is generally associated with extractions of the terminal tooth in the maxilla, usually the third molar. An isolated, over-erupted second or third molar represents a particularly dangerous situation and a fracture is extremely likely. It can be prevented by palpating the alveolar bone during extraction, removing locking buccal bone and, if necessary, sectioning the tooth.

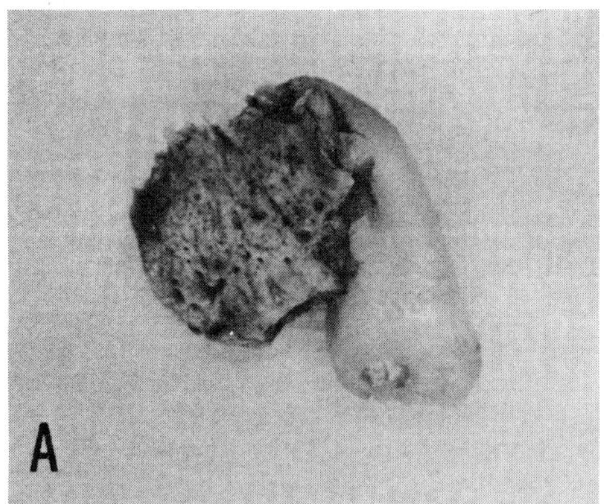
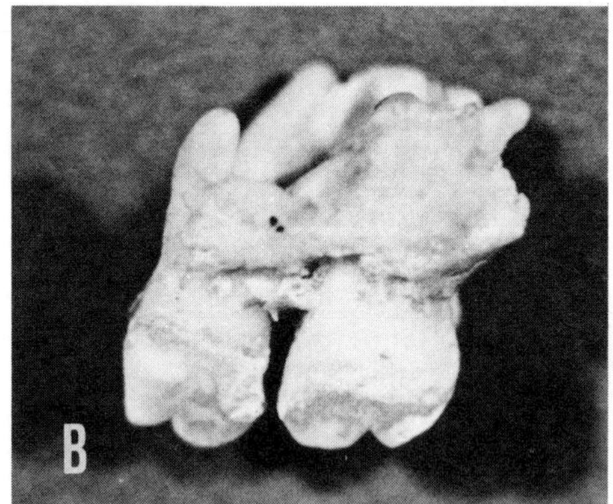

Figure 5.A. Fracture of tuberosity asociated with third moral extraction. B. Ankylosis of second and third molars resulting in severe tuberosity fracture. (Courtesy of Col. Robert M. Huey).

Treatment

If the tuberosity does fracture, a few suggestions may prove useful:

- **If motion is slight and the segment small, section and remove the tooth leaving bone segments attached to the periostium.**
- **If severe with a large segment of bone involved:**
    a. Stop the extraction and equilibrate the tooth.
    b. If the tooth is partially extracted, section the crown and leave the roots in place. Remove the roots after the tuberosity is no longer mobile, usually in six weeks.
    c. If necessary, splint the tooth so the fracture will heal.

Loss of the tuberosity is a serious complication from the prosthodontic viewpoint. Surgically, it is rather easy to manage simply by primary closure of the wound margins. A massive fracture involving the maxillary sinus, can result in a defect difficult to compensate for prosthodontically. In addition, if the sinus is involved, immediate surgical management is much more complex and referral to an oral surgeon is indicated.

STUDY EXERCISE

Four things you can do to help control the amount of bone loss during routine exodontia in the maxillary arch are:

a. ____

b. ____

c. ____

d. ____

The primary concern in the posterior area of the maxillary arch is the location of the maxillary _____________________ *and the maxillary* _____________________

The use of excessive force during the extraction procedure may fracture a _____________ *or* ____.

By placing your thumb and index finger on each side of the maxillary alveolus in the maxillary pinch grasp position it is possible to both:

a. _____________________*the alveolus.*

b. _____________________*any abnormal movement of the bone.*

IF BONE IS REMOVED WITH A TOOTH it should be examined, then (replaced/discarded) _____________________. *Any jagged*_____________________*left by the fracture should be*_____________________*with rongeurs or a bone file. Soft*_____________________*is then repositioned to*_____________________*close the extraction site, ESPECIALLY if the portion of bone at the apex of the tooth may have involved the sinus floor.*

IF A FRACTURE IS DISCOVERED BEFORE THE BONE IS REMOVED FROM THE SOFT TISSUE, you should________________________the bone from the _________________________ without displacing the________________and its________________supply. This may be done by careful elevation or sectioning of the tooth. You (should/should not) ____________ _______________reflect a flap over the fractured area. This will________________the bone fragment and________________its chance for survival. With the tooth removed, the bone fragment may be positioned and supported by________________.

If a large fracture develops, especially in the tuberosity, you should _________________ the procedure and________________________the teeth.

If the tooth is partially extracted,________________the crown and________________ the roots. After the tuberosity is stable, usually after ________________________ weeks, you would remove the roots.

FRACTURE OF THE MANDIBLE

One of the most dramatic complications is fracture of the mandible during tooth extraction. This is almost always avoidable, and is most frequently caused by carelessness. It is most commonly associated with removal of a moderately deep, vertically impacted third molar.

Prevention

This problem is usually due to excessive force with an elevator. Preventive measures include careful evaluation of radiographs and careful use of elevators. It is usually wise, when removing an impaction, not to attempt any technique for the removal of the tooth or portions of the tooth that rely on expansion of the bone to achieve tooth movement. You should realize that in this area of the mandible, with the thick cortex of the oblique ridge, the amount of cancellous bone which can be compressed is minimal. It is best to use a bur or chisel to create space.

Treatment

Mandibular fractures occurring in this manner are routinely treated with reduction and intermaxillary fixation. It is wise to refer them to an oral surgeon.

NOTE: Treatment of mandibular fractures should be referred to an oral surgeon unless you have had special training in this area. Serious occlusal problems may result from an inadequately managed fracture of the mandible.

Preventive measures to reduce possible mandibular fractures include:
1.________________ ________________of   radiographs.
2.________________use of an elevator.
3. Use of a technique that (does/does not)________________require the expansion of bone.

INJURIES TO ADJACENT TEETH

Possible complications involving the adjacent teeth include:

- **Partial avulsion**
- **Fracture of cusps, incisal edges, or restoration.**
- **Extraction of the wrong tooth.**

Beware of the "crowded tooth trap." Removal of a tooth between two overlapping teeth requires a high level of skill to avoid loosening, avulsing, or fracturing incisal edges of adjacent teeth.

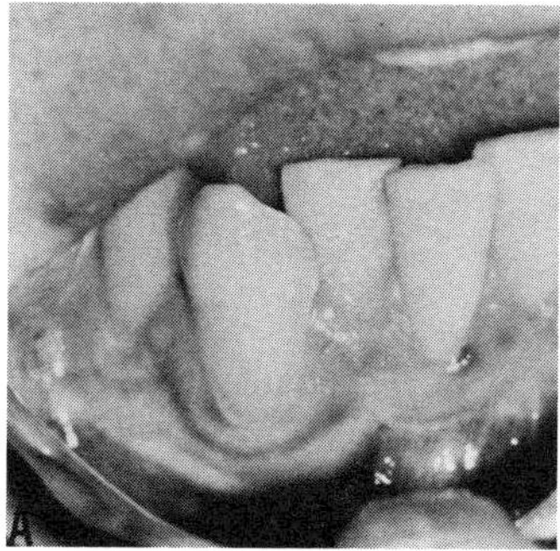
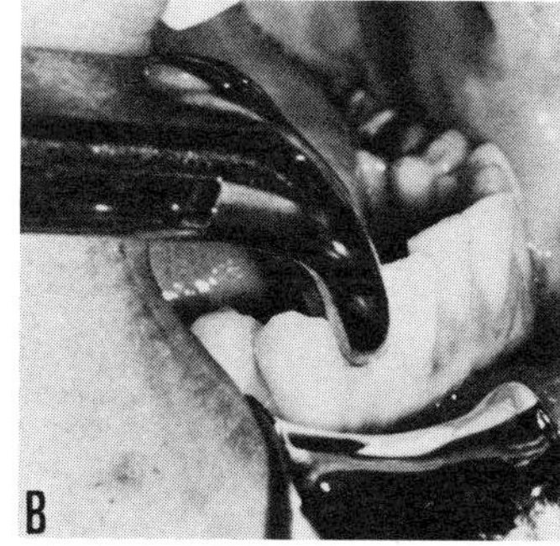
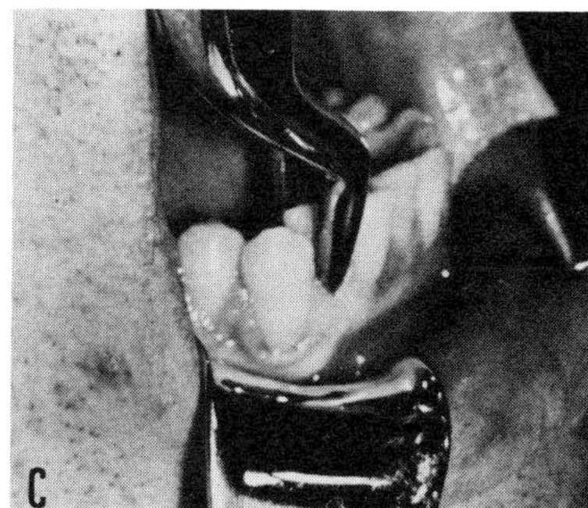

Figure 6. A. A lateral incisor which is overlapped. B., Application of a 151 forceps. Note that the forceps is too wide and will damage the adjacent teeth. C. Application of 286 forceps. The beaks are narrow enough to permit labial-lingual movements without damage to adjacent teeth.

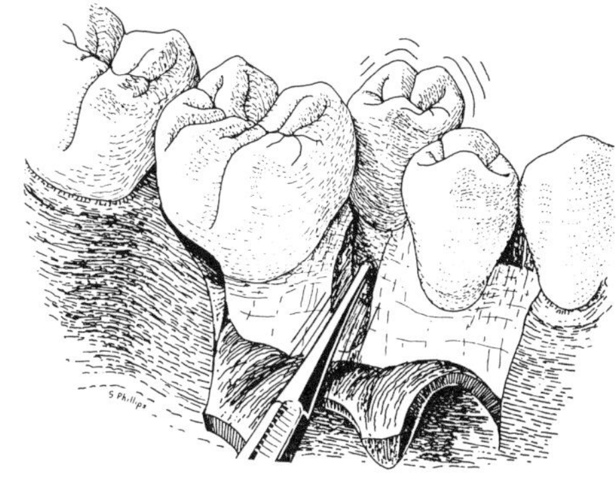

Figure 7. In the event that no forceps can be adapted to the tooth, or when a forceps can be adapted but no movement is possible without disturbing the adjacent teeth, the so-called "broken instrument technique" should be employed. A flap is reflected on the buccal-labial aspect and a small amount of bone is removed, permitting access to a point just apical to the cervical line. A shallow purchase point (hole) is established and a fine-bladed elevator or the end of a broken hand instrument is inserted into the purchase point. A few sharp, light taps will effect delivery of the tooth. (Howe, 1971).

Partial Avulsion of the Adjacent Tooth

Loosening of adjacent teeth occurs either with improper placement of an elevator or trying to use an inappropriate forceps.

Treatment

If the tooth is loosened, it should be stabilized with either a wire or acrylic splint. If it has been completely avulsed, it should be re-implanted and then stabilized. Endodontic therapy should be planned for any tooth that has been completely avulsed. During stabilization the tooth should not be in occlusion so that trauma is minimized during the healing process.

Fracture of Cusp, Incisal Edges, or Restorations

The fracture of an incisal edge is almost always preventable. However, many large amalgam restorations and underextended crowns and inlays on the distal of the first and second molars represent "disasters waiting to happen." Amalgams are frequently poorly condensed and have insufficient retention. It will be a sizable challenge to remove the second or third molar without damaging these restorations. Transmission of any force to these restorations can result in dislodgement.

Prevention

Fractured cusps usually occur in adjacent teeth that have extensive restorations (especially second molars during an attempt to remove impacted third molars). Thus, in these situations, you should try to avoid placing any instruments against these adjacent fillings, and do not put heavy leverage force against them. You should also avoid forces which will push the tooth being extracted up against the adjacent filling. It is necessary to warn the patient in advance of the probability of restoration fracture.

Treatment

When a fracture of a tooth or restoration does occur, a temporary filling material should be placed **AFTER** completion of surgery. The patient should be informed of the problem and plans made for complete replacement of the filling. If a crown or an inlay has been displaced, it can be re-cemented **AFTER** the surgery has been completed. Care should be taken, however, that the temporary filling material or the cement does not fall into the extraction socket where it can cause a foreign body reaction.

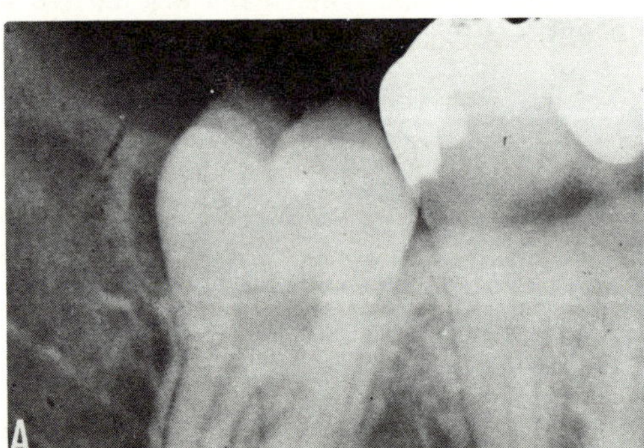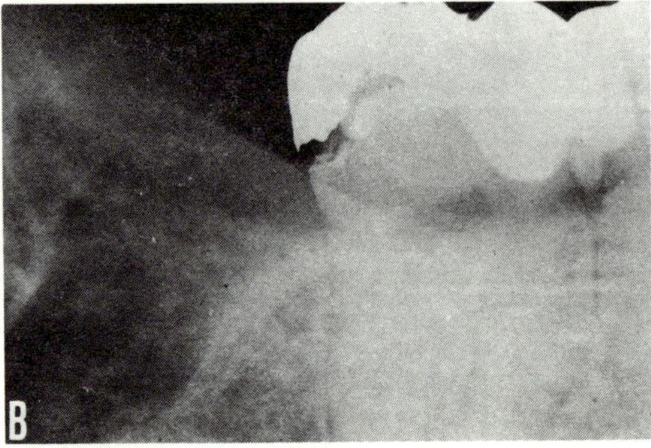

Figure 8. A. X-ray of impacted tooth. Note MOD inlay in second molar. B. Inlay has been dislodged by the third molar as it was elevated from its socket. (Courtesy R. C. Gordon, D.D.S., M.S.).

STUDY EXERCISE

Three possible injuries to adjacent or other teeth that can occur during an extraction procedure are:

1. ____

2. ____

3. ____

Fracture of cusp tips or restorations should be treated in the following way:

____

____

____

What should you tell your patient before surgery concerning possible fracture of cusp tips or restorations?

____

____

____

Extraction of the Wrong Tooth

When performing extractions for your own patients there is little danger of extracting the wrong tooth since you are responsible for the treatment plan. But, when referring a patient to an oral surgeon, who is essentially performing prescription surgery, or in treating your own patient who is referred to you by an orthodontist, there is danger of improper communication or of indicating the wrong tooth for extraction on the referral form. In both instances there is ample room for error. Special precautions are indicated.

Prevention

Removal of the wrong tooth for orthodontics can be avoided by checking with the orthodontist if any doubt exists, and by marking the teeth prior to the procedure with an indelible pencil. It is a good practice to have your assistant confirm the treatment plan just prior to removal of the tooth.

NOTE: Removal of the Wrong Tooth Does Occur Often Enough that You Should Always be Aware of the Possibility and Take Special Steps to Avoid it.

Treatment

When the wrong tooth is removed, it should be replaced as rapidly as possible and stabilized until healing occurs. Plans must also be made for endodontic therapy. In the case of the removal of premolars prior to orthodontic treatment, it may be wise to check with the orthodontist if you find that you have accidentally removed the wrong tooth. In some cases the orthodontist may be able to revise the treatment plan and accommodate this mistake. As unpleasant as the task may be, it is imperative that the patient and the orthodontist be informed of what has happened as soon as possible.

STUDY EXERCISE

Extraction of the wrong tooth usually occurs for two reasons:

1. ____
2. ____

COMPLICATIONS ASSOCIATED WITH INDIVIDUAL TOOTH REMOVAL

Fractured Roots

Fracture of roots and root tips is a common problem. Generally all fractured roots should be removed, however, you must weigh the degree of surgery required to remove a tip with the possible consequences of leaving the tip in place.

Prevention

Before removal of any tooth, a close examination of periapical radiographs will reveal any condition that may increase the possibility of a fractured root during extraction. You should be suspicious of any of the following conditions:
(1) Slender roots
(2) Curved roots
(3) Divergent roots
(4) Ankylosed roots (teeth in which the periodontal ligament space cannot be seen)
(5) Devitalized teeth
(6) Dense alveolar bone

Although any of the above factors could increase the likelihood of fracturing a root during surgery, the major cause of fractured root tips is the improper use of instruments, such as forceps or elevators.

NOTE: Following Extraction of any Tooth, the Roots Should Be Examined For Evidence of a Fractured Root Tip.

Displaced Teeth

Teeth or Roots Displaced into the Maxillary Sinus.

It is possible to displace maxillary teeth into the maxillary sinus either during forceps extraction or root retrieval. The tooth most commonly affected is the conically rooted, partially erupted maxillary third molar. When attempting to extract this tooth with forceps, the forceps may slip, "shooting" the tooth into the sinus. If you believe a significant risk exists for displacing a tooth into the maxillary sinus, the tooth should be removed surgically, using an elevator for appropriate direction of force.
It is quite easy to displace roots of molar teeth into the maxillary sinus.

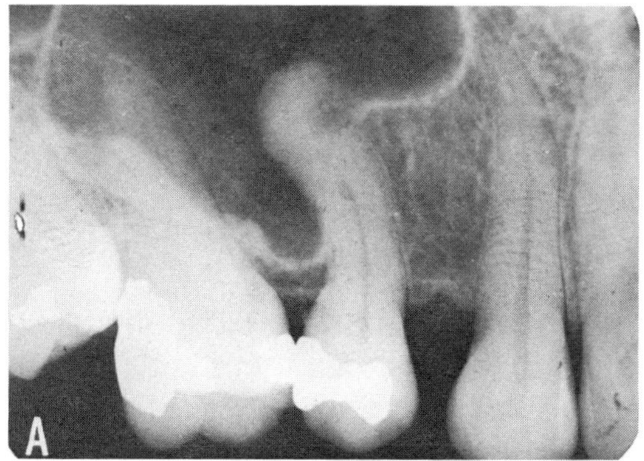
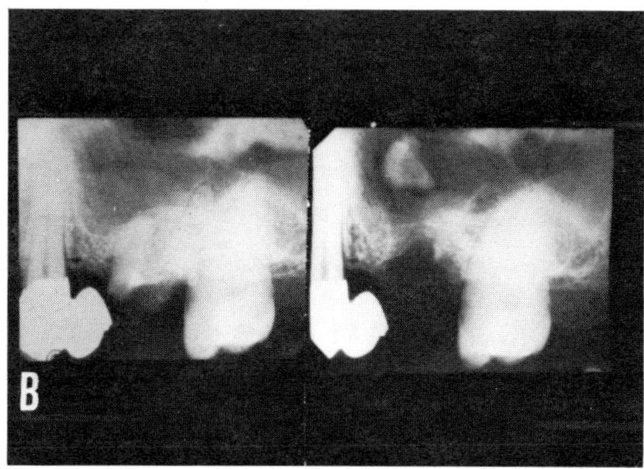

Figure 9. A. Root vulnerable to maxillary sinus displacement. B. Palatal root of first molar displaced into maxillary sinus. (Courtesy of J.R. Hayward, D.D.S., M.S.).

The root most easily dislodged into the sinus is the palatal root of the first molar. It is always safer to extract such a root surgically by approaching the socket laterally via a flap raised in the buccal sulcus. If you attempt to remove maxillary molar roots without laying a flap, you risk forcing the root or elevator into the maxillary sinus.

Prevention
A careful pre-operative assessment should alert you to the hazard of pushing a root tip into the maxillary sinus. The usual conical shape of the maxillary third molar and the thinness of the bone in the tuberosity region make it quite easy to displace the tooth into the sinus or the infra-temporal fossa. The patient should be informed of this possibility before the extraction. Displacement of the maxillary third molar into the sinus usually occurs when the surgeon does not get the elevator above the height of contour of the tooth before pressure is applied.

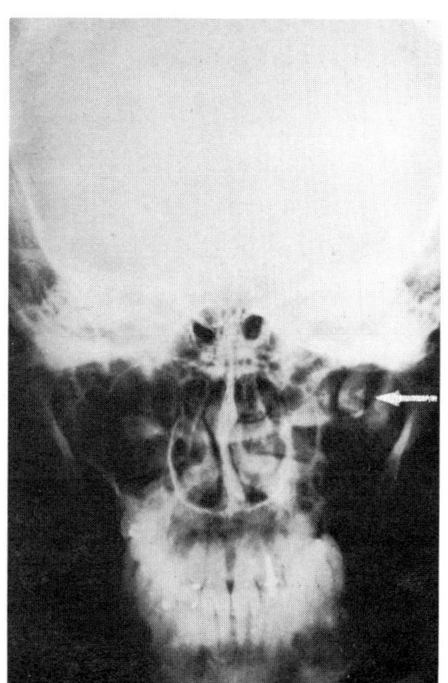

Figure 10. Maxillary third molar displaced into pterygomaxillary space, right side of radiograph. (Courtesy of J.R. Hayward, D.D.S., M.S.).

Treatment
If the root is "lost" and thought to be in the sinus, surgical intervention is delayed until it is established radiologically that the root is in the sinus and not simply lying subperiostally or between the sinus membrane and bone.

You should not attempt to remove a root tip (or tooth) from the sinus **through the extraction socket** as this may **increase** the likelihood of **sinus infection** and/or **oro-antral fistula formation.** You should close the wound (as disclosed on pages 30 through 32) and **refer the patient to an oral and maxillofacial surgeon for removal of the root tip.** A surgeon will remove the root tip via a Caldwell-Luc approach through the canine fossa, which reduces the possibility of oroantral fistula formation.

Teeth or Roots Displaced Into Soft Tissue Spaces

The lingual plate of bone in the third molar region of the mandible usually is extraordinarily thin, especially in the apical region. In many instances there is a fenestration of the bone with a direct communication into the submandibular space. This must be taken into account in any effort to remove a mandibular third molar, especially when the tooth is sectioned with a chisel, or when small root tips are being retrieved. There have been many reported cases of teeth that have actually been pushed into the submandibular space during attempts to remove a third molar.

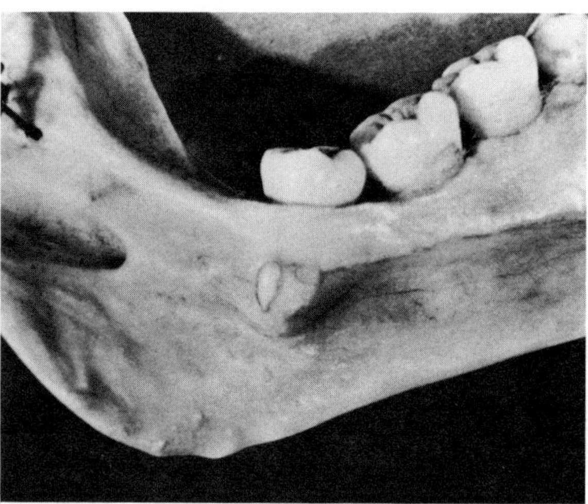

Figure 11. Lingual surface of mandible. Note the fenestration in the region of the third molar roots. It is easy to see how the roots could be pushed into the submandibular space.

Prevention

When attempting to section an impacted mandibular third molar, it is a sensible precaution to place one finger over the lingual plate of the bone in order to prevent the tooth from being pushed into the submandibular fossa.

A more frequent problem is that of pushing a small root tip through the lingual plate of bone while attempting to retrieve the root tip. When the bone is fenestrated, this would seem to be an almost unpreventable complication. Extreme care should be used in attempting to retrieve a lingually posed third molar root tip. It is a wise procedure to place a finger over the lingual plate of bone so that you can feel the root tip as it begins to enter the submandibular space.

Treatment

When a root tip has been displaced into the submandibular space beneath the mylohyoid muscle, you should thoroughly evaluate the situation before attempting to remove it. It would be wise to spend approximately ten to fifteen minutes in an effort at retrieval. A conservative approach of attempting to palpate the root tip beneath the periostium and manipulate it back into the socket should be tried at this time. If this is not successful, the patient should be advised of the presence of the root in the submandibular space and referred to an oral surgeon for evaluation.

Not all root tips in the submandibular space have to be removed. In evaluating the situation, the oral surgeon will weigh the possible effects of retrieval versus potential ill effects of leaving them. A fractured root that has been forced through the lingual plate is usually removed utilizing a large mucoperiosteal flap from the alveolar ridge on the lingual side of the mandible and recovering the root with small curved curettes. This is facilitated by the use of extraoral counter pressure over the involved area to prevent additional displacement of the root during manipulation of the tissues.

STUDY EXERCISE

Fracture of roots may be minimized by:
1. Close examination of____.
2. Proper use of____.

State the greatest difficulty that an operator may get into when removing impacted third molars.

____

____

Maxillary third molars or their roots are occasionally displaced into:
a) ____
b) ____
Mandibular third molars are occasionally displaced into:
a) ____

If a tooth has been displaced into surrounding tissue, you should:

____

____

____

Now re-take Pre-test, Unit II, and progress as indicated.

UNIT III

OTHER INTRA-OPERATIVE COMPLICATIONS

Complications associated with the maxillary sinus
    Opening into the maxillary sinus
    Oro-antral fistula
Temporomandibular joint injury
    Trauma
    Dislocation of the condyle
Broken Instruments
    Broken needles
    Broken elevator tip

PRE-TEST FOR UNIT III

- *Cover answers on Page 29.*
- *Answer the following questions.*
- *Check your answers against those on Page 29.*
  If all are correct, proceed to Unit IV.
  If you got some of the answers wrong, turn to Page 30 and begin Unit III.

Questions:

1. *How is the temporomandibular joint stabilized during the extraction of a tooth?*

2. *If the patient complains of temporomandibular joint pain immediately following surgery, what should you do?*

3. *During an inferior alveolar nerve block, the needle suddenly breaks off at the hub and disappears into the soft tissue. How is this treated?*

4. *While you are using a 301 elevator to remove root tips from a mandibular third molar, the tip of the elevator suddenly disappears into the socket. On aspiration you cannot find the tip of the elevator. What should you do?*

5. *Describe how you would evaluate if a patient has an oro-antral communication following extraction of a maxillary posterior tooth. If one is detected, what is the treatment?*

6. *What should you do if a patient develops chronic sinusitis and an oro-antral fistula following removal of a maxillary molar?*

PRE-TEST — UNIT III, Answers

1. *With either a sling support or a bite block.*
2. *Place the patient on a soft diet and warn him not to open his mouth wide. Provide analgesics and advise him about moist heat for the area to make it comfortable.*
3. *Refer the patient to an oral surgeon as soon as possible.*
4. *Take an x-ray to locate it.*
5. *The nose-blowing test. If opening is less than 2 mm, no closure is necessary. An opening greater than 2 mm should be closed using a surgical flap.*
6. *Establish drainage, irrigate, prescribe antibiotics. If the sinusitis does not respond to this therapy, refer to an oral surgeon.*

CONTENTS FOR UNIT III

OTHER INTRA-OPERATIVE COMPLICATIONS

COMPLICATIONS ASSOCIATED WITH THE MAXILARY SINUS

Opening into the Maxillary Sinus

The maxillary sinus is closely related to the roots of the maxillary posterior teeth (Figure 12). The pre-operative radiographs can show the relationship of the sinus to the roots of the teeth. When the roots of the teeth are indented into the sinus, then oro-antral communications are frequently produced when extracting these posterior teeth (Figure 13).

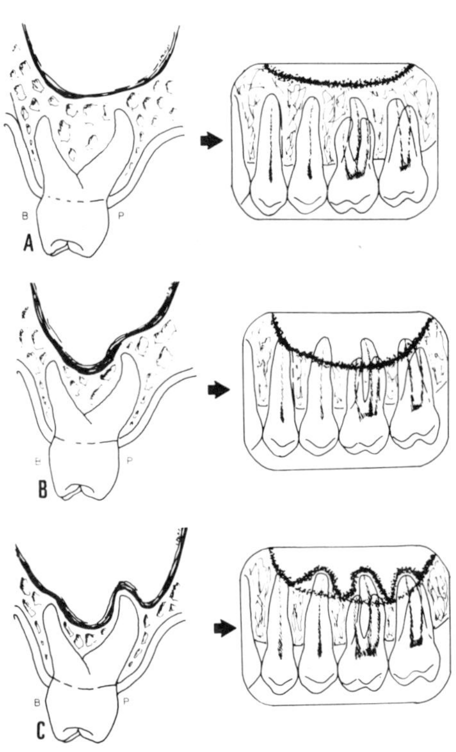

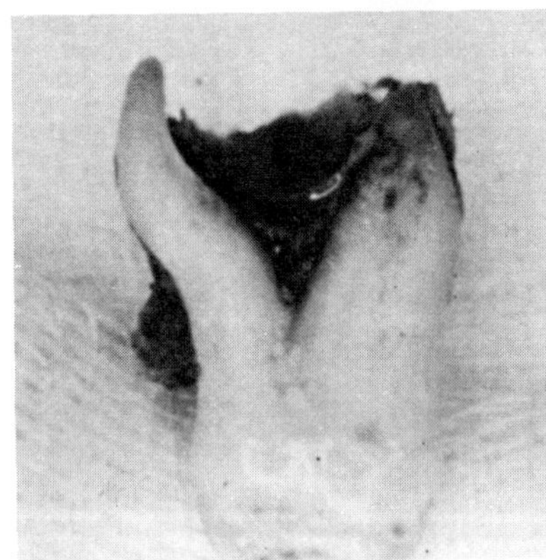

Figure 12. X-ray assessment of maxillary first molars. A. The roots are not closely related to the maxillary sinus. B. The roots of the first molar appear to be piercing the sinus but are actually located bucally and palatally to the sinus. C. The roots of the first molar actually protrude into the floor of the maxillary sinus. Note the normal lamina dura around the apex of the roots.

Figure 13. Floor of sinus adhering to maxillary first molar.

Some authors suggest probing of the sockets in order to determine the presence of a communication, but this practice can introduce oral flora into the sinus or can create an opening where none existed. A better method is the nose-blowing test. The nose is squeezed and the intranasal pressure is increased, producing a whistling noise that may be heard as air passes down the defect.

If the presence of a communication is confirmed, its size should be determined. If the opening is two millimeters or less, a surgical closure is not necessary providing an adequate blood clot forms and is retained for organization and healing. For larger openings, a flap should be designed to close the defect.

To prevent sinusitis, an antibiotic, such as penicillin-V, is prescribed for five days. In addition, the use of a decongestant nasal spray is suggested with instructions to spray the appropriate nostril every four hours in order to keep the osteum patent and encourage normal sinus drainage.

It is important that the patient not inadvertently dislodge the blood clot from the socket of the extracted tooth. It is necessary to be thorough in reviewing post-operative instructions and to warn the patient against increasing intra-sinus pressure by nose blowing and sneezing or negative oral pressure such as sucking on straws or smoking.

If the opening into the maxillary sinus is **greater than two millimeters**, and it appears that the blood clot probably would not be retained, a surgical flap is necessary (Fig. 14). The flap is designed to include the surgical area. It is usually necessary to reduce buccal bone to allow the flap to approximate the palatal tissue. To increase the elasticity of the mucoperiosteal flap, the periosteum must be incised near the base of the flap. In approximating the flap, it is necessary to have a slightly everted suture line to get maximum contact of the wound edges. As with any oro-antral communication, antibiotics and decongestants are prescribed.

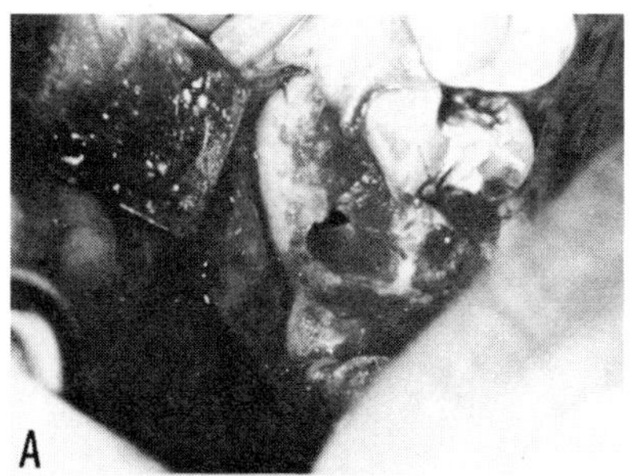
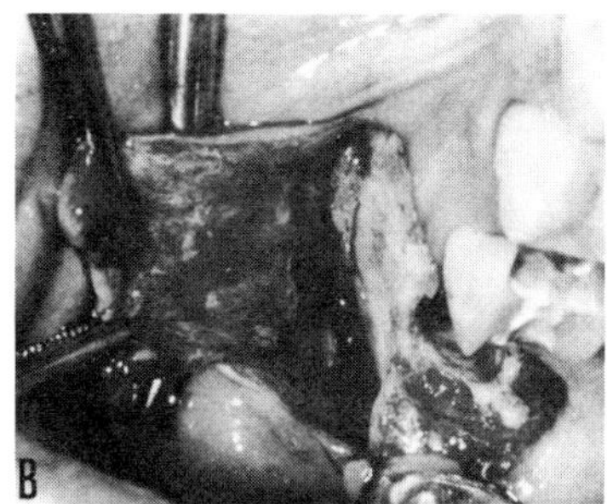
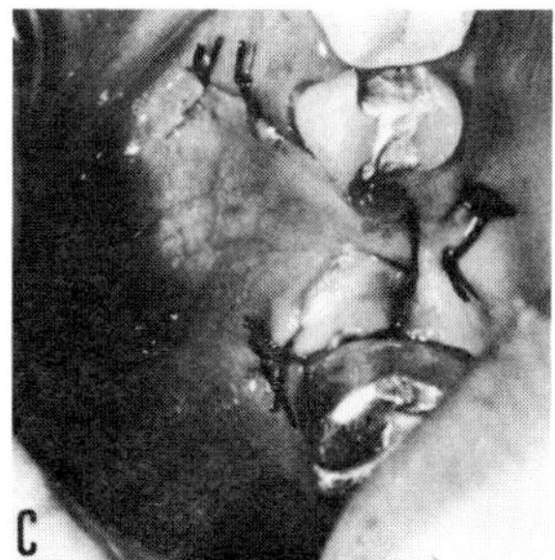

Figure 14. Technique for immediate closure of oro-antral communication. A. Note communication at base of distobuccal root of maxillary first molar. B. Mucoperiosteal flap reflected. Note that the periosteum has been incised horizontally at the base of the flap to allow it to stretch across the socket. C. Mucoperiosteal flap sutured.

Oro-antral Fistula

As pointed out by Shira (1972), most tooth socket openings between the oral cavity and the maxillary sinus (oro-antral communications) will heal spontaneously. When there is an acute or chronic sinusitis present or when the opening is enlarged, an oroantral fistula may develop (Fig. 15). These fistulas should be closed. Their treatment is generally considered to be in the realm of the oral surgeon.

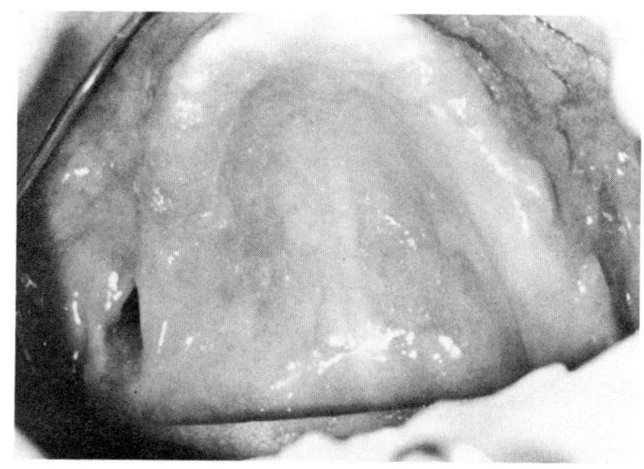

Figure 15. Chronic oro-antral fistula in the maxillary second molar region.

Treatment

The first step in the treatment consists of an attempt to clear up the sinus infection. This is achieved by establishing drainage, irrigation, and by antibiotic therapy. If the sinusitis does not respond to conservative treatment, it will be necessary to perform a Caldwell-Luc operation in which access to the sinus is gained through the canine fossa. The diseased antral mucosa is stripped away and an additional opening, a nasal antrostomy, may be made into the nasal cavity for improved drainage.

After the sinus infection is resolved, it is possible to close the oro-antral fistula. A number of techniques have been advanced for this purpose. The most popular is the use of the buccal flaps outlined in Figure 14. Since this flap has to stretch over the defect, it frequently results in a decrease in vestibular height in the affected region. In situations where this would cause a severe prosthodontic problem, it would be advisable to consider a palatal flap to close the wound.

A common cause of failure of oro-antral fistula repair is acute maxillary sinusitis. To prevent this, these patients are generally placed on prophylactic antibiotics and a decongestant nasal spray to maintain good nasal drainage.

STUDY EXERCISES

If you suspect an oro-antral communication following extraction of a maxillary molar, how would you confirm this? ____

____

How would you treat oro-antral communications in the following cases?
Communication is less than or equal to 2 mm ____________________________________
Communication is greater than or equal to 2 mm __________________________________

What medications and special postoperative instructions would you give a patient if you discover an antral communication? ____________________________________

____

How would you treat a patient who develops an oro-antral fistula? _________________

____

TEMPOROMANDIBULAR JOINT INJURY

Trauma

Trauma to the temporomandibular joint capsule usually occurs when the mandible is improperly supported during routine exodontia procedures. Since there is no anatomical support against the lateral forces used routinely in exodontia, all the forces used during the extraction are transferred directly to the temporomandibular joints. Fortunately, the patient will usually complain of pain from the joint area when the mandible is not being properly supported. However, there are some cases in which the patients do not have pain, or at least do not complain about it during the procedure.

Prevention

Stability of the temporomandibular joint can be provided with a sling support of the mandible or use of a bite block. With difficult extractions of mandibular molars, you may find that no matter how well you support the mandible, the patient still will complain of pain in the temporomandibular joint. In this case, it is wise to resort to surgical removal of the tooth.

Treatment

If there is temporomandibular joint pain immediately following surgery, you should place the patient on a soft diet and instruct him not to open his mouth wide. Analgesics, such as aspirin, can be provided along with moist heat to make the joint area more comfortable.

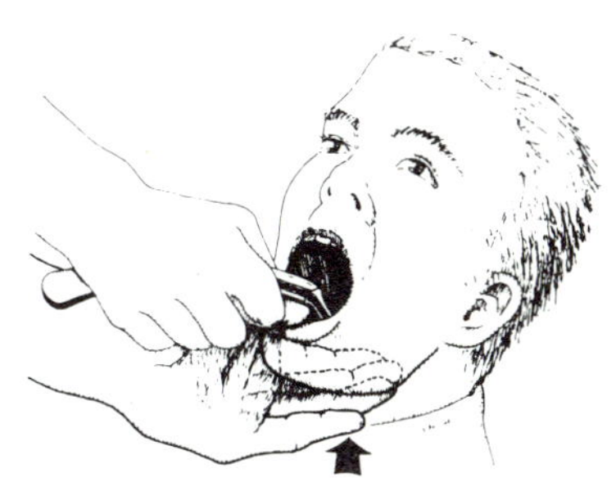

Dislocation of Condyle

A more acute problem during mandibular extractions may be the dislocation of the condyle from the glenoid fossa.

Prevention

This can be prevented by using the same precautions listed on page 33.

Treatment

This problem should be immediately corrected by standing behind the patient, placing your thumbs on the external oblique ridge of the mandible, and rotating the posterior portion of the mandible downward and forward.

NOTE: If you place your thumbs on the occlusal surface of the teeth, you may be injured as the teeth snap into occlusion during the reduction of the dislocation.

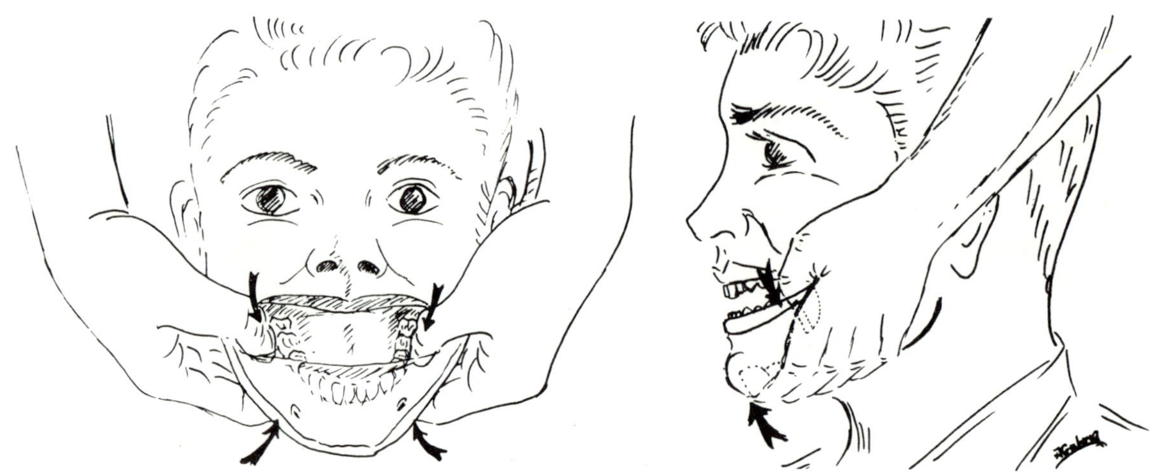

Broken Instruments

Broken Needles

If syringe needles are reused, they become weakened and may break off in tissues during an injection. This complication rarely occurs now, as compared to a few years ago, with the advent of disposable needles.

Prevention

By routinely using disposable needles you will avoid this complication.

Treatment

If the needle breaks off inside soft tissue and is not easily retrievable, it is best to refer your patient to an oral surgeon for a decision as to whether it is necessary to remove the needle. There is some debate as to whether leaving broken needles would cause problems. This type of decision should be left to one more experienced in the surgical procedure of removing the needle.

Broken Elevator Tips

Elevator tips can fracture when used with excessive force. This usually occurs when using straight elevators, such as number 301 or 34.

Prevention

Use of controlled forces with elevators should reduce the possibility of this complication.

Treatment

Irrigate and debride the region and then attempt to find the metal fragment. If it cannot be found readily, take a radiograph to locate it. If you still can't find it, refer the patient to an oral surgeon.

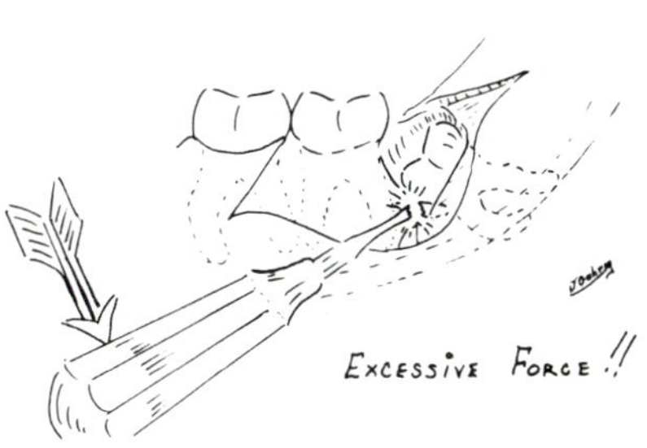

Do not use excessive force when using elevators

STUDY EXERCISE

If a needle should break off inside soft tissue you should __________________________

____

Should you break an elevator tip, you should:
1. ____
2. ____

Now re-take pre-test, Unit III, and proceed as indicated.

CONTENTS FOR UNIT IV

POST-OPERATIVE CARE

Appropriate patient education
  Bleeding
  Swelling
  Discomfort
  Diet
  Medication
  Oral hygiene
  Sleeping and physical activity

APPROPRIATE PATIENT ECUCATION

Appropriate patient education can be a very important step in preventing post-operative complications. You should verbally supplement your written instructions. Advise your patients to contact you if they have any questions or problems during the post-operative period. Include your emergency telephone number. This will allow you to discover and treat any complications early. The forms on Pages 38-39 demonstrate a sample post-operative form presented to surgical patients. You should orally review and discuss the following points with your patient.

Bleeding

Remind the patient that the gauze should be kept in place for one hour post-operatively. Instruct the patient on how to place a dampened gauze pack over the extraction site if there is any further bleeding.

Swelling

If the patient has had a soft tissue flap reflected, especially if there was any bony surgery, strong emphasis should be placed on the use of ice packs applied to the side of the face over the operated site. Emphasis should be on immediate application of ice packs and, if necessary, an ice pack may be made available to the patient before he leaves the office. Ice packs should be used only on the day of surgery. **Instruct the patient not** to apply heat to the area because this will increase swelling.

Discomfort

Inform the patient that the greatest discomfort is usually experienced when the anesthetic wears off. Instruct the patient to take the initial dose of any analgesic prescription **before** sensation returns to the area. The medication is less likely to control post-operative pain if postponed until discomfort is severe.

Diet

Instruct the patient that a high protein, soft diet with high fluid intake is desirable. To encourage adequate diet during convalescence, food supplements such as the liquid diet foods and instant breakfast are suggested.

Medication

Analgesic, antibiotic, and sedative medications should be prescribed as indicated. You should fully instruct your patient in the proper method of taking the medications and, if necessary, write out the instructions in longhand before the patient leaves.

Oral Hygiene

Emphasize that the patient should avoid vigorous rinsing of the mouth or spitting for the first twelve hours following surgery. The patient can be reassured that after this period he can carefully brush his teeth and tongue in areas away from the sites of surgery. After 24 hours, he can also rinse his mouth carefully to prevent debris from accumulating around the extraction or surgical site. The patient can be told to resume normal brushing of the teeth in the area of surgery whenever it becomes comfortable or at least within five days.

Sleeping and Physical Activity

Encourage the patient to rest for at least 24 hours. This is especially true if any bone has been removed or a periosteal flap elevated.

STUDY EXERCISE

What postoperative instructions will you give your patients concerning the following subjects?

Bleeding ____

Swelling ____

Discomfort ____

Diet ____

Medications ____

Oral Hygiene ____

Sleeping and Physical Activity ____

POST-OPERATIVE TREATMENT
(Sample Form)

Thank you for coming to the School of Dentistry for your oral surgery treatment. Your treatment continues until healing is complete. Therefore, please call your student, who is ________________________________, at phone number________________________________, who will arrange for emergency service if necessary.

THINGS TO EXPECT:

Swelling: This is normal following a surgical procedure in the mouth. It should reach its maximum in 24 to 48 hours and diminish by the fourth post-operative day.

Discomfort: The most discomfort you will experience will be during the period when sensation returns to your mouth.

Hemorrhage: Bleeding or "oozing" for the first 12 to 24 hours is to be expected.

THINGS TO DO:

1. Bleeding. Bite on the sponges placed in your mouth at the end of the procedure for at least one hour. If bleeding is more than slight, follow these directions: with gauze, remove all excess blood clot. Place a dampened gauze over the bleeding area only. Hold this pack in place firmly for twenty minutes, so that no blood escapes. Repeat this procedure as necessary. Call the student on call if the bleeding persists.

2. Swelling. The swelling that is normally expected is usually in proportion to the surgery involved. This swelling may be minimized by the immediate use of ice or cold packs. Apply ice to the side of the face over the operated site. Place pack on face for fifteen minutes, and then remove for fifteen minutes. Continue for a few hours. Prolonged use of ice is of no value.

3. Diet. After waiting one hour, one should be able to take fluids by mouth. A liquid or soft diet may be necessary for the first two days. This would include soups, soft drinks, cereals, mashed potatoes, etc. An adequate fluid intake of at least two quarts a day is essential.

4. Medications. Take all medications as directed. This is essential. The medications are prescribed principally to control pain and to prevent infection.

5. Mouth Rinse. Do not rinse on the day of surgery. Rinsing the mouth with warm salt water—one teaspoon to an 8-ounce glass—following meals is advisable. This will speed healing by maintaining a clean wound.

THINGS NOT TO DO:

1. Do not apply heat to the face at any time. This will increase the swelling.

2. Avoid spitting. This creates a negative pressure in the mouth and tends to dissolve the blood clot—in turn, this leads to additional hemorrhage.

3. Avoid strenuous physical activity for twenty-four hours. This includes bowling and swimming and other sports in which one becomes winded. Physical activity causes the blood pressure to rise—and may cause a renewal of the hemorrhage.

IMPACTED TEETH: The removal of impacted teeth is quite different from the extraction of erupted teeth.

The following conditions are not uncommon with removal of impacted teeth.

Difficulty in opening your mouth
Pain while swallowing
Earache on the side of surgery

If a lower impaction was removed, you may have numbness of the lower lip on the side from which the tooth was removed. This is almost always a temporary condition. It is not disfiguring, just annoying. It may last from a few days to many months.

After removal, the adjacent teeth may realign themselves, causing some discomfort.

Sores may develop at the corners of the mouth. These should be covered with a mild ointment (Vaseline).

In the event that you feel that your post-operative course is marked by excesses of pain, swelling, or hemorrhage, do not wait for your next appointment. Call the student at the number listed.

UNIT V

POST-OPERATIVE COMPLICATIONS

Hemorrhage
  Health history screening for bleeding problems
  Planning surgery
  Following surgery
  Controlling hemorrhage
Fibrinolytic alveolitis
  Prevention
  Treatment
Bone spicules
Nerve injuries
  Inferior alveolar nerve
  Lingual nerve
  Mental nerve

PRE-TEST FOR UNIT V

- *Cover answers on Pages 42-43.*
- *Answer the following questions.*
- *Check your answers against those on Pages 42-43.*
  If all are correct, proceed to next unit.
  If you got some of the answers wrong, turn to Page 44 and begin Unit V.

Questions:

1. *State the reasons why the patient's answer to each of the following questions will be helpful in alerting you to potential bleeding complications:*
   a. *Have you ever had liver disease?*

   b. *Do you have hypertension?*

   c. *Do you bruise easily?*

   d. *Has anyone in your family had a history of bleeding problems?*

2. *Why is a prothrombin time important?*

3. *Why is a partial thromboplastin time an important test?*

4. *Why should the surgeon attempt to remove all granulation tissue during a surgical procedure?*

5. *What are the most common vessels encountered in routine oral surgery?*

6. *Why does one usually not have to worry about injury to the nasopalatine artery and vein?*

____

7. *What steps can you take in treating the patient before he leaves your office that can prevent many post-operative bleeding problems?* ____________________________

____

8. *If the patient returns to your office in the middle of the night with the complaint of excessive blood loss, what are three things that should be evaluated:*
    (a) ____
    (b) ____
    (c) ____

9. *During the examination of an extraction site that had excessive blood loss post-operatively, you notice a single small point of bleeding from the distal portion of the bony socket. What is your treatment?*______________________________________

____

10. *During the examination of a patient presenting for post-operative hemorrhage, you find that the blood welling up in the socket is coming from multiple areas within the socket. Pressure does not seem to control the hemorrhage. The evaluation of the patient's clotting ability shows him to be normal. What is your treatment?*

____

____

11. *During surgical removal of an impacted maxillary canine, you note one area of blood spurting from the palatal flap. The blood vessel is deep within the flap, so that it cannot be clasped with a hemostat. How would you handle it?*

____

____

12. *List three clinical signs and symptoms of fibrinolytic alveolitis.*
    (a) ____
    (b) ____
    (c) ____

13. *List at least four things that have been implicated as possible causes of fibrinolytic alveolitis.*
    (a) ____
    (b) ____
    (c) ____
    (d) ____

14. *How will you treat fibrinolytic alveolitis?* ________________________________

____

15. *If you know that the inferior alveolar canal is close to the roots of an impacted third molar, what steps should you take to avoid injuring the nerve?*
    (a) ____
    (b) ____
    (c) ____

16. *During what steps in the removal of the mandibular third molar can the lingual nerve be damaged?* ____

____

17. *When laying a flap around the mental foramen, what steps should you take to avoid injuring the nerve?* ____

____

18. *Two weeks after the removal of a mandibular third molar, the patient reports to your office with sharp spicules protruding from the surgical area. What is your treatment?*

____

PRE-TEST — UNIT V, *Answers*

1. a. *There are six clotting factors that are produced in the liver.*
   b. *A high diastolic blood pressure could mean abnormal pressure that may break down a normal clot.*
   c. *This may be a symptom of a patient who has a disease involving platelet formation or capillary fragility.*
   d. *There are multiple bleeding disease that are congenital.*
2. *It will pick up most of the defects in the extrinsic portion of the clotting system.*
3. *It will pick up the majority of the hereditary clotting disorders.*
4. *Because the high vascularity of the tissue may cause post-operative bleeding.*
5. *The inferior alveolar, mental and the greater palatine blood vessels.*
6. *Hemorrhage is a very rare problem with this group of vessels.*
7. *Have the patient remain in the chair for an extra fifteen minutes after surgery and change the gauze or pack just prior to his leaving the office to determine if the bleeding is under control.*

8. *(a) Blood loss, (b) patient's present physical condition, (c) the reason for the hemorrhage.*
9. *Attempt to burnish the bone with the tip of a hemostat.*
10. *Use one of the local hemostatic substances such as Gelfoam, Oxycel, or Surgicel.*
11. *Attempt to stick-tie by encircling the vessel and the surrounding tissue with a suture, tying tightly.*
12. *(a) Lost blood clot, (b) extreme pain, (c) halitosis with a complaint of bad taste in the mouth.*
13. *Any of these six: excessive trauma; poor blood supply; infection; infiltration nerve blocks; extensive use of mouth rinses; poor oral hygiene.*
14. *Carefully irrigate the socket with warm water under local anesthetic if necessary and carefully pack the socket with strips of iodoform gauze and medicated dressing. This dressing should be changed after the first 24 hours and then every two days for a period up to ten days.*
15. *(a) Inform the patient of the possibility of anesthesia. (b) Take care to prevent undue trauma to the nerve, especially when using a bur. (c) Observe extreme care while curetting the socket, especially at this depth.*
16. *During the original incision that is carried too far lingually and, when the tooth is being sectioned with a bur, by carrying the bur to the lingual cortex.*
17. *Carefully identify the mental foramen before proceeding with the surgery.*
18. *These most likely are sequestrated bone bits and should be carefully removed with a hemostat or curette under local anesthesia.*

UNIT V

POST-OPERATIVE COMPLICATIONS

INTRODUCTION

Post-operative complications are those that can occur after the patient leaves the office. The management of post-operative pain and infection is described in another chapter. Hemorrhage, fibrinolytic alveolitis, and nerve injuries will be described in this unit.

HEMORRHAGE

In most cases post-operative hemorrhage tendencies can be detected before the patient leaves your office by having the patient remain in the office for 15 minutes after you have completed your procedure. This routine, along with a good health history and proper planning, will prevent a great majority of hemorrhage problems.

Health History Screening for Bleeding Problems

A health history for screening these potential problems should include the following questions:

✔ **Have You Ever Had an Episode of Prolonged Bleeding?**
This question can be expanded by also asking such questions as:

Have you experienced prolonged bleeding following dental extractions?

If you have ever cut yourself, has it taken longer than ten minutes to control the bleeding?

If you have had any surgery, has the surgeon mentioned that he had difficulty controlling the bleeding?

(If the patient is a woman.) Have you experienced any bleeding difficulty associated with childbirth or during menstrual flow?

✔ **Have You Had Liver Disease?**
This question is helpful since all of the blood clotting factors, except Factor XIII, are produced in the liver. Other variations of this question are:

Have you ever had hepatitis?

Have you ever been jaundiced or yellow?

How much alcohol do you drink daily?

⌐ Do You Have Hypertension (High Blood Pressure)?
Excessive hypertension does not influence the clotting factors but may cause profuse bleeding. The patient's diastolic pressure is most important here, since it corresponds closely with the relatively constant pressure at the capillary level. Although any diastolic pressure above 90 mm Hg is considered abnormal, a pressure above 120 mm Hg should be considered as a contraindication to even minor surgical procedures.

NOTE: A DIASTOLIC PRESSURE GREATER THAN 120 MM Hg SHOULD BE CONSIDERED A DEFINITE CONTRAINDICATION TO EVEN MINOR SURGICAL PROCEDURES.

⌐ Are You Presently On Any Anticoagulant Therapy?
Presently there seems to be an increase in the use of anticoagulants for various medical problems. Until recently, the most frequent indication for the use of anticoagulants was a history of myocardial infraction or cerebral vascular accident. Anticoagulant therapy for these conditions is now questioned by many cardiologists.

The current absolute indications for anticoagulation therapy include: prosthetic heart valves; deep venous thrombosis; pulmonary embolus; other thromboembolic phenomena.

Variations of this question are:

Are you presently taking any medications?

Are you taking any medications to "thin down" your blood?

Have you recently experienced a heart attack?

Have you ever had heart surgery?

Have you ever had any thromboembolic phenomena? (Explain)

⌐ Do You Bruise Easily?
A patient who bruises easily may have a disease involving platelet formation or increased capillary fragility. When the possibility exists, a bleeding time should be ordered. The standardized normal Ivy bleeding time is an accurate method.

⌐ Do You Have Anemia?
Depending upon the severity of the anemia, a patient may have difficulty withstanding even small amounts of blood loss.

It is unwise to perform elective surgery on patients who have or are suspected of having anemia.

✔ Has Anyone in Your Family Had a History of Bleeding Problems?

There are many genetic disorders which result in either decreased amounts of certain coagulation components, ineffective coagulation components, or both. It is not unusual to encounter patients with undiagnosed coagulation disorders. **Hemophilia A** is the most common inherited coagulation disorder representing about 1/20,000th of the general population. Approximately 30-40% of newly diagnosed hemophiliacs have no previous family history of hemophilia. Therefore, these patients may present without a confirmed diagnosis. In addition, patients who suffer from mild disorders of coagulation (e.g. von Willebrand's) may not have had sufficient stress placed on their coagulation system to demonstrate an abnormality. Therefore, on occasion, you may discover these disorders following a surgical procedure.

The question with regard to a history of bleeding problems in the family is very important, but as the above information points out, a negative answer does not guarantee absence of a genetic bleeding disorder.

STUDY EXERCISE

What routine, following surgery, will greatly reduce your post-surgical bleeding problems? ____

Taking a good health___________________, and proper___________________will also decrease your frequency of post-operative complications.

In a health history screening of the patient before performing surgery, you would want to ask the following questions to detect potential bleeding problems:

a.____
b.____
c.____
d.____
e.____
f.____
g.____

Regarding potential hemorrhage, why should you know if the patient has had liver disease? ____

What problem would be caused by hypertension?_______________________________

A diastolic pressure of greater than ___________mm Hg should be considered a definite contraindication to even___________________________________surgical procedures.

Two reasons a patient may be on anticoagulant therapy are:

1. ____
2. ____

Four absolute indications for anticoagulant therapy are:

1. ____
2. ____
3. ____
4. ____

Bruising easily may be a sign that your patient may have a disease involving:

1. ____
2. ____

A patient with anemia will be (more/less)_____________________able to tolerate surgery that involves excessive blood loss than a healthy patient.

Two hereditary blood disorders that your patients may have are:

1. ____
2. ____

Do patients generally know if they have a serious bleeding disorder? Yes _____, No _____.

Planning Surgery to Minimize Hemorrhage

The second important step in preventing post-operative hemorrhage is careful planning of any surgical procedure you may undertake. The following four rules should be followed in this respect:

> ✔ **Know the Reason for any Previous Bleeding Problems That Have Been Uncovered in the Health History**
> This may be a very simple task if the patient has some hereditary clotting defect that has been well documented. If, however, the patient has had no previous documentation of clotting deficiencies, it is necessary for you to determine if the patient truly has a bleeding problem, and if he does, refer him to a physician for care. There are a group of four blood tests that can rule out any potential bleeding problem.

Platelet Count

This test detects both thrombocytopenia and thrombocytosis. Both can cause a prolonged bleeding time. It should be pointed out that a platelet count will give only an indication of the number of circulating platelets present at that time. It has no bearing upon the function of those platelets. Certain disorders such as von Willebrand's disease or aspirin ingestion can decrease the functional capacity of the platelets without changing the absolute number. Therefore, a platelet count will indicate only half of the picture.

Prothrombin Time

This test will pick up defects in the extrinsic portion of the clotting system. These would include Factor V, Factor VII, Factor X, prothrombin and fibrinogen. A deficiency in any one of these factors is usually due to an acquired disease. A common example is:

Liver Disease

All clotting factors with the possible exception of Factor XIII are synthesized in the liver. Liver diseases (e.g., cirrhosis) appear to more commonly affect the Vitamin K dependent factors, e.g., prothrombin. The Vitamin K independent factors, e.g., fibrinogen, plasma thromboplastin antecedent may be synthesized in adequate amounts even in chronic liver disease.

Partial Thromboplastin Time

This test detects most defects in the whole blood clotting process, but it is primarily a test of the intrinsic system involving Factors VIII, IX, XI, and XII.

Bleeding Time

This test detects von Willebrand's disease, the third most common hereditary disorder. The standardized Ivy method, generally the preferred test, can be performed by placing a blood pressure cuff immediately above the elbow and inflating it to 40 mm pressure. Using a template, a small cut is made in the forearm with a disposable lancet, and the time required for the blood to clot is measured. The normal value is 5 minutes ± 2 minutes.

Surgical Technique

By following the precautions below during surgery, you will reduce post-surgical hemorrhage problems in your patients.

✔ Remove All Granulation Tissue

The presence of highly vascularized granulation tissue makes the control of hemorrhage difficult.

✔ Do Not Tear or Crush Tissue

A bleeding vessel is readily seen on a sharply dissected flap. But, if the tissue has been torn, the bleeding vessel may be almost impossible to locate. Crushing the tissue causes multiple areas of hemorrhage, which are difficult to control.

✓ Know the Anatomy of the Surgical Area

Knowledge of anatomy is especially important in respect to the position of any major vessel. The most common vessels encountered in routine oral surgery are:

- Inferior alveolar vessels with their continuation into the mental vessels, and

- The greater palatine blood vessels.

A dentist who plans to reflect extensive flaps should also know the position of the lingual and facial vessels, since both can be encountered in the oral cavity. One should also be aware of small vessels in the lingual portion of the mandibular incisal area and the lingual portion of the retromolar area. One does not usually have to worry about the nasopalatine artery and vein, since hemorrhage from this group of vessels is very rarely a problem.

STUDY EXERCISE

Four simple tests that can be performed by a dentist to rule out any bleeding problem are:
1. ____
2. ____
3. ____
4. ____

Granulation tissue should be eliminated because_____________________________________.

Why should sharp incisions be used in reflecting soft tissue flaps? _______________
____

What two rules should be adhered to in the planning for oral surgery?
1. ____
2. ____

Controlling Hemorrhage Following Surgery

After the surgery is completed, there are steps that can be taken to prevent post-operative hemorrhage problems. The first is to ensure that bleeding is under control before the patient leaves the office.

NOTE: YOU CAN DETERMINE IF BLEEDING IS UNDER CONTROL BY HAVING YOUR PATIENT REMAIN IN THE OFFICE FOR 15 MINUTES FOLLOWING SURGERY, AND THEN CHANGING THE GAUZE PACK JUST PRIOR TO THE PATIENT'S DEPARTURE.

Careful planning and presentation of post-operative instructions can be of help in reducing the number of late night calls from patients with bleeding problems. Your patients should be instructed to maintain pressure on the gauze for 45 to 60 minutes after the procedure. Show them how to place dampened gauze over the extraction or surgical site if bleeding continues. They can also be warned to expect blood-tinged saliva for 24 hours after surgery. However, your patients should feel free to give you a call if hemorrhage persists.

Controlling Post-Operative Bleeding
When a patient returns to your office with a complaint of excessive hemorrhage, it is imperative that you make a full evaluation in respect to:

- Amount of blood loss

- Present physical condition

- Reason for hemorrhage

Blood Loss

The estimation of the amount of blood loss can be obtained by careful questioning. It is common that a patient will tell you that he or she is able to fill a container of a certain size, or that a certain number of gauze sponges have been used. You can estimate the blood loss by figuring at least 75% of any volume as actual blood loss, or that a 2x2 gauze sponge absorbs about 2.5 cc of blood. An adult patient who has lost in excess of 500 cc of blood should be referred to an oral surgeon, or, if that is not possible, to a local hospital.

Present Physical Condition

The patient's over-all condition can be quickly assessed by noting whether he exhibits any weakness and whether he shows signs of shock. The classic signs of shock include:

- Hypotension
- Increased breathing rate (hyperpnea)
- Pallor
- Cold sweat
- Thirst
- Restlessness
- Weak and rapid pulse

Reason for Hemorrhage

After you have assessed the patient's condition, you can determine the source of hemorrhage. This should be initially attempted WITHOUT LOCAL ANESTHESIA. Use of local anesthetic may obscure the point of bleeding. After the exact area of hemorrhage is determined, an INITIAL attempt to control hemorrhage should be made with moist gauze sponges and pressure. In the majority of cases, this is all that is necessary.

STUDY EXERCISE

If you determine that a patient has lost in excess of_____________cc of blood, you would most likely refer him to an oral surgeon or hospital. How can the volume of blood loss be determined? ____

____

____

What do you look for in determining a patient's over-all condition? ________________

____

If you find the patient's condition satisfactory and blood loss minimal, what would be your initial plan to control the problem?

____

____

What steps, initiated after surgery but before the patient leaves the office, can be taken to minimize post-surgical bleeding problems?
a. Ensure that____before the patient leaves the office.
b. Instruct the patient to__________________________for ____________________ following the procedure.

If your initial attempt to control hemorrhage with pressure is not successful, then local anesthesia should be given and the following methods used to control the problem locally. When possible, nerve blocks should be used instead of infiltrations, if you wish to find the point of hemorrhage. The vasoconstrictor in the local anesthetic may stop the hemorrhage. This is a technique that is used by some practitioners to control hemorrhage, but does have a disadvantage in that the hemorrhage may be only temporarily controlled until the vasoconstrictor is metabolized.

STUDY EXERCISE

If you administer local anesthetic when attempting to control hemorrhage you should use _____________________________ rather than _____________________________.

Methods of Controlling Hemorrhage From Bone

If careful examination of the surgical site shows that the bleeding is from the bone, then one of the following three procedures can be applied.

Crushing or Burnishing the Bone

This can best be done with the tip of a hemostat if there are small, single points of bleeding. When there are multiple points of hemorrhage so that you cannot determine the individual source vessels, this method will be of little help.

Absorbable Sponges

These local hemostatic substances can be best used in bony defects, such as extraction sockets. The substances form a matrix on which the clot can build, and may provide support for platelets, even when there is a defect in the prothrombin or fibrinogenic phase of coagulation. The commercial products that are available include Gelfoam and Surgicel. It must be emphasized that these sponges control hemorrhage only by providing a clotting matrix and cannot be used for pressure dressings.

Bone Wax

This substance is not usually stocked in dental offices, and therefore is rarely used in oral surgical procedures. It is effective in stopping extensive bleeding from extraction sockets, especially if the inferior alveolar artery or vein has been violated. The big drawback in the use of bone wax in the tooth socket is that it is poorly absorbed and may contribute to post-operative infection.

Following examination, you determine that a patient's bleeding problem is due to hemorrhage from bone. What options for treatment do you have?

1. _______________________________________

2. _______________________________________

3. _______________________________________

For each of the following situations state which method of controlling bone hemorrhage would be best:

1. A small single point of bleeding in the lateral wall of the socket from which a tooth has been removed.

____

____

2. Multiple small bleeding points in an extraction socket.

____

____

3. Extensive bleeding from inferior alveolar artery following removal of a deep impaction.

____

____

What is the big drawback to this method? _______________________________________

Soft Tissue Bleeding

The following methods can be used if the hemorrhage has been localized to the soft tissue.

Pressure

Pressure is applied to slow the flow of blood, permitting clotting to take place. The use of a moist gauze sponge has been previously described as the most common method used in oral surgery. If a flap has been reflected, it is sometimes helpful to replace or add sutures to control the bleeding. An acrylic splint, such as an immediate denture, can also provide pressure enough to stop bleeding. However, this is only helpful when the splint has been constructed pre-operatively.

Tying Vessels

Individual bleeding vessels can be controlled either with a CLAMP TIE or a STICK TIE. When the vessel is exposed in a position such that a small hemostat can be placed on the end of it, it is relatively easy to place the ligature around the vessel. The ligature used in the oral cavity is plain gut of either 3/0 or 4/0 size.

It is rare in the oral cavity to come across a vessel that can be easily clamped. In most cases it is necessary to proceed to a STICK TIE, which is accomplished by encircling the vessel and surrounding tissue with the suture. The suture is then tied in hopes of occluding the vessel.

Clamp Tie   **Stick Tie**

STUDY EXERCISE

Soft tissue bleeding may be controlled by_______________or______________ _____________ ____ .

Pressure can be used to control hemorrhage and is used in the following way: _________ ____ ____

Tying vessels may be necessary. Two methods are____________tie and____________tie. When one can occlude the cut end of a small vessel, the_________________tie method is preferable; when not, the_________________tie method must be used.

FIBRINOLYTIC ALVEOLITIS

A new term, **"fibrinolytic alveolitis,"** used to describe what has more commonly been called **alveolar osteitis**, or **dry socket**, has been suggested by Birn. Fibrinolytic alveolitis is without doubt the most common post-operative problem encountered in exodontia.

The clinical appearance of this disease is well known. Two or three days after removal of the tooth, the blood clot disintegrates. The alveolus is empty with completely or partially denuded, very sensitive bone surfaces covered by a grayish-yellow layer of detritus and necrotic tissue. The surrounding gingiva often shows an inflammatory reaction. The patient complains of violent pain, usually throbbing in character, which radiates toward the ear and the temple region. Halitosis is pronounced, and the patient complains of a bad taste in the mouth. Swelling of the regional lymph nodes is rather common. General symptoms such as increased temperature are seldom seen, but the patient may be physically affected because of severe pain and feel unwell due to lack of sleep and appetite.

The etiology of "FA" (fibrinolytic alveolitis) has been illustrated by Birn's series of investigations. They reveal that FA develops because of high fibrynolytic activity in and around the alveolus. This gives rise to the dissolution of the blood clot and the formation of kinins, which cause the violent pain in this disease. In this way, the two most important characteristics in FA are explained by a common pathogenesis. Fibrynolytic activity arises from the alveolar bone around the wound by release of stable tissue activators. It is well known that tissue activators are liberated by inflammation in the tissue. Heavy inflammation of the marrow spaces is characteristic of FA. The inflammation is most probably caused by infection of the alveolus or trauma. These are the two most probable causes of FA. While fibrynolysis is the provoking factor in FA, infection as well as trauma may be the etiology of the disease.

There are many conflicting opinions as to the importance of the two factors in the etiology of FA. This may be due to the fact that one has been more pronounced than the other in individual cases. Infection and trauma may work together to create the degree of inflammation which is necessary for the development of FA.

The etiology and pathogenesis of FA are explained diagrammatically in Figure 15. Infection and trauma cause inflammation of marrow spaces of the alveolar bone. This gives rise to liberation of tissure activators which convert plasminogen in the blood clot to plasmin. This dissolves the blood clot and at the same time releases kinins from kininogen, which is also present in the clot. The final result will be dissolution of the blood clot and violent pain.

It is quite unusual to have FA following a routine extraction. Extensive clinical investigations have shown that the disease develops in 2.0 to 4.4% of all extractions of permanent teeth. The incidence in the mandibular third molar region has been reported to range from 0.9 to 62.5% with the average approximately 30%. Since the incidence of FA is so high following third molar removal, it is incumbent upon you to do whatever possible to prevent this most unpleasant complication.

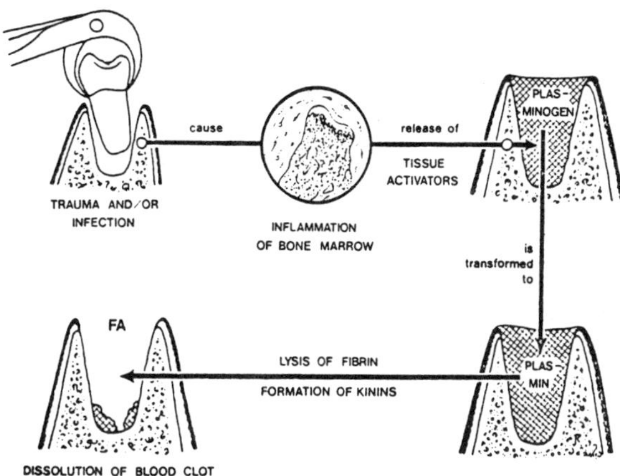

Figure 15. Etiology and pathogenesis of fibrinolytic alveolitis. (From H. Birn, "Etiology and Pathogenesis of Fibrinolytic Alveolitis," *Int J Oral Surg, 2:252,* **1973, with permission).**

Prevention

In the absence of a scientific method of prevention, a number of empirical suggestions can be made:

- Trauma should be kept to a minimum. Careful surgical procedures should be carried out rather than the indiscriminate use of force.
- The wound should be carefully debrided.
- Nerve blocks rather than infiltration should be used in the third molar region.
- A broad spectrum antibiotic such as tetracycline, used topically in the socket, may decrease the incidence of FA.

Treatment

FA is not a progressive disease and will persist from 10 to 14 days whether treated or not. The therapeutic goal is to relieve the patient's discomfort. Treatment for FA is:

- Irrigate the debris from the socket using at least 200 cc of warm saline solution. This may be so painful during the first treatment session that administration of a local anesthetic should be considered.

- Following irrigation, the socket area is isolated from saliva by using cotton rolls or gauze.

- A medicated dressing on plain or idoform gauze is inserted. The following is a formula for a typical dressing:

    Eugenol 46%
    Balsam of Peru 46%
    Chlorobutanol 4%
    Benzocaine 4%

The dressing should be applied loosely in the socket, covering all of the exposed bone.

Typically, the dressing is changed after the first 24 hours and then every other day during the first week. During the second week of treatment, when the pain generally becomes less intense, the dressing can be left in place for three to four days at a time. It is unusual to have to dress the socket for more than two weeks. If this is necessary to obtain pain relief, the patient should be thoroughly re-evaluated to ensure that osteomyelitis does not develop. After analgesics are not required systemically, the dressing should be discontinued since it may mechanically retard repair.

STUDY EXERCISE

The term FIBRINOLYTIC ALVEOLITIS is a more accurate term for ___________________
______________________*or*___________________   ___________________.

The clinical appearance of FA includes:
a. ____
b. ____

What steps can be taken to minimize the chances of a patient developing this problem?
a. ____
b. ____
c. ____
d. ____

*How would you treat fibrinolytic alveolitis?*_________________________________
____

BONE SPICULES

After removal of a tooth your patient will sometimes complain of pieces of bone coming out of the socket or sticking out of the gum in the area of the surgery. This is common when the sockets have not been carefully debrided following the surgical procedures. These bits of bone are dead and in most cases they do not cause any problem except discomfort to the patient. It is usually easy to remove the spicules with a hemostat or curette under local anesthesia. It is rare for these bone particles to cause any form of infection, although they may contribute to secondary infection of the area.

NERVE INJURIES

Nerves are rarely directly visualized during an oral surgical procedure; thus the first symptoms of nerve injury are not recognized until the post-operative period. A few nerves in the oral cavity, however, are routinely sacrificed without consequence: specifically, the nasopalatine and the long buccal nerves. These nerves are sensory to such small areas that most patients are not aware of a change in sensation. The inferior alveolar, the lingual, and the mental nerves do pose a problem in oral surgery and care should be taken not to damage them.

Inferior Alveolar Nerve

Before removing any impacted mandibular third molar, the relationship of the mandibular canal to the tooth should be determined. If it appears that the canal is so near the third molar that it may be damaged during removal of the tooth, the patient should be warned before the surgery of possible consequences.

During the procedure, care should be taken to prevent undue trauma to the nerve, especially when using a bur to divide the tooth. While curetting the socket, be careful of any soft tissue present at the depth of the socket. Most commonly, the nerve is "bruised" when the apex of the third molar brushes against it. This injury causes only minor damage and the nerve recovers completely within one to two weeks.

The possibility of complete severance of the mandibular nerve is fortunately very low. When this does occur, it is wise to replace the severed portions of the nerve within the canal and assure that there is no obstruction. In many cases this will allow the proximal end of the severed nerve fibers to regenerate along the canal and achieve some amount of reinnervation. However, this may take up to six months.

Lingual Nerve

Damage to the lingual nerve can occur during routine dental injections, or during the removal of the mandibular third molar. Injury during injections, however, is quite rare, especially considering the number of inferior alveolar blocks given. During third molar surgery, the nerve can be violated by either carrying the bur through the lingual cortex while attempting to divide a tooth, or by placing the initial incision too far lingually. When damage to the nerve is evident, the chances are that sensation will return within a few weeks. However, this is not always so. If sensation does not return within three months, a referral should be made to an oral surgeon experienced in neurorrhaphy (nerve repair).

Mental Nerve

Prevention of damage to the mental nerve is probably the easiest of the three major nerves because the nerve can be visualized and avoided during the surgical procedure. When reflecting a flap in the area of the mental foramen, an attempt should be made to identify the foramen and its contents as soon as the flap has been elevated. Obviously, care should be taken to avoid the nerve when any vertical incision is made in this region. Once this bundle has been identified, retraction can be used to carefully protect the nerve from damage during the surgical procedure.

However, you should also realize that the mental nerve cannot tolerate much tension and has been shown to divide during even mild retraction. The chances for return of sensation, if this nerve is severed, are small.

STUDY EXERCISE

Which nerves in the oral cavity are routinely sacrificed without consequence?
a. ____
b. ____

Which nerves in the oral cavity should the surgeon take care NOT to injure?
a. ____
b. ____
c. ____

One prime consideration during the assessment of difficulty of removal of an impacted mandibular third molar is injury to the inferior alveolar nerve.
a. *What do you tell the patient concerning potential problems?*_______________
____

b. *During the procedure, what can you do to minimize undue trauma to the nerve?*
____

c. *What is the most common cause of inferior alveolar nerve damage during impaction surgery and how long does this damage usually affect the nerve?* _______________
____

d. *What do you do if you know that the nerve has been severed during your procedure?*
____

How should one attempt to minimize trauma to the mental nerve?
a. ____
b. ____

How much force of retraction can this nerve tolerate? _______________________

If severed, what is the potential for return of sensation? ___________________

If bone spicules should remain following the removal of teeth:
1. *What problem may this cause the patient?* _______________________________
____

2. *What should be done about it?* _______________________________________
____

How may the lingual nerve be damaged during impaction surgery?
a. ____
b. ____

What would you tell the patient who has no sensation in one side of the tongue two days after a mandibular extraction? _______________________________

*What do you do if sensation DOES NOT return within a few weeks?*_______________

POST-SURGICAL PAIN

While pain is a normal post-operative occurrence, pain can become a surgical complication if it exceeds the level of analgesia you have prescribed. Since the amount of pain perceived by a patient can vary from individual to individual, you should:
- Plan the management of post-operative pain prior to beginning surgery (review each patient's past history of pain).
- Plan your surgical procedure to anticipate and minimize intra-operative complications.
- Obtain adequate anesthesia in the surgical area (intra-operative pain can excite your patient to higher levels of post-surgical pain).
- Use a long-acting local anesthetic to allow your patient to obtain their post-surgical analgesic before the anesthetic dissipates.
- Minimize the time required for surgery.
- Prescribe "adequate" analgesics to the level of surgery performed, and present your analgesic prescription to the patient in a positive manner.

While a complete discussion of post-surgical pain control is beyond the scope of this book, you should always keep in mind that **inadequate post-surgical pain control can cause unnecessary patient distress and increase the frequency of "after-hours" complaints.**

POST-SURGICAL INFECTION

When performing surgery in the mouth, the risk of post-surgical infections (both oral and systemic) must always be considered. Measures **can be taken** to reduce the probability of post-surgical infections (e.g. good aseptic technique; reducing oral flora, plaque, and calculus; careful wound debridement; etc.). Careful post-surgical monitoring of patients can allow you to detect post-operative infections early and facilitate prompt and effective management or referral. The diagnosis and management of post-surgical infections is discussed in greater detail in other books in this series.

SUMMARY OF SURGICAL COMPLICATIONS

POTENTIAL COMPLICATIONS	PRE-SURGICAL EVALUATION AND PLANNING	PRECAUTIONS DURING SURGERY	MANAGEMENT
SOFT TISSUE INJURIES			
Mucosal tear	Plan adequately-sized flaps.	Reflect flaps carefully.	Suture the wound.
Puncture		Use controlled force with elevators (and other instruments).	Irrigate the wound. Closely follow the patient's healing.
Inadvertent incision		Pay careful attention to scalpel and incision site during surgery.	Suture the wound if deep.
Heat injuries	Instruct auxiliaries to check that all instruments are cool prior to surgery.	Check new instruments placed on tray during surgery.	Apply vaseline. Evaluate for scarring when healed.
Abrasion and avulsion		Retract the lip when using rotary instruments.	Palliative treatment.
Crush injuries		Keep lips out of way (not over teeth with instruments on top).	Palliative treatment.
BONE FRACTURE			
Fracture of the maxillary alveolus	Evaluate x-rays for relationship of roots to the maxillary sinus.	Use a "pinch grasp." Use controlled force. Remove buccal or labial bone when indicated (e.g. labially positioned cuspid, isolated maxillary molar). Section teeth if indicated.	If bone is attached to periosteum: do **not** lay flap. Remove the tooth, reposition bone, and suture to support while healing. If bone has been separated from soft tissue: smooth jagged edges of bone; position and suture soft tissue to cover exposed bone or antral openings.
Maxillary tuberosity fracture	Beware of an isolated super-erupted posterior tooth	Section teeth if indicated. Remove buccal bone.	If segment is small, carefully remove teeth. For large segment, equilibrate the tooth and splint tooth to allow bone to heal.

POTENTIAL COMPLICATIONS	PRE-SURGICAL EVALUATION AND PLANNING	PRECAUTIONS DURING SURGERY	MANAGEMENT
Fracture of mandible	Evaluate x-rays.	Do not rely on bone expansion in molar area. Use adequate bone removal (especially in mandibular 3rd molar area).	Refer to oral and maxillofacial surgeon for intermaxillary fixation.
DAMAGE TO ADJACENT TEETH			
Partial avulsion	Recognition of problem, instrument selection, indication for referral, advise patient of risk.	Adaptation of technique and/or instrument selection.	Stabilize tooth with wire and acrylic splint and reduce occlusion. Reimplant and stabilize if completely avulsed; plan endodontic treatment
Fracture of tooth or restoration	Evaluate proximity of adjacent teeth and **warn patient of potential problems.**	Avoid leveraging against adjacent teeth and restorations.	Place a temporary restoration after completing surgery.
Extraction of the wrong tooth	Confirm surgery request with orthodontist.	Have assistant confirm treatment plan immediately prior to extraction. Mark tooth with indelible pencil.	Replace and stabilize tooth. Plan endodontic therapy. Consult orthodontist.
DAMAGE TO TOOTH BEING EXTRACTED			
Fractured root	Evaluate radiographs for: slender, curved or divergent roots; devitalized teeth; dense bone; ankylosed teeth; referral.	Properly elevate teeth prior to forceps use. Remove bone and/or section tooth if indicated.	Remove surgically.
Displacement into maxillary sinus	Evaluate radiographs for relationship of roots to sinus.	Remove bone and/or section teeth if indicated.	Refer to an oral and maxillofacial surgeon.
Displacement into the submandibular space	Recognize increased risk when removing partially erupted or fully impacted mandibular 3rd molars.	Place finger over lingual plate while sectioning a mandibular tooth or removing a root tip. Use care when retrieving root tips; don't push apically.	Attempt to manipulate root back into socket. If unsuccessful, refer to an oral and maxillofacial surgeon.

POTENTIAL COMPLICATIONS	PRE-SURGICAL EVALUATION AND PLANNING	PRECAUTIONS DURING SURGERY	MANAGEMENT
MAXILLARY SINUS			
Opening into the sinus (non-epithelialized oroantral communication	Evaluate radiographs for relationship of roots to the sinus.	Use surgical technique (flaps and tooth/root sectioning) to reduce risk. Do not probe socket after extraction.	**If 2 mm or less,** closure is not necessary. Instruct patient not to dislodge blood clot (no smoking, nose-blowing, suction, etc.)
			If greater than 2 mm, design a surgical flap for primary closure and prescribe antibiotics. Recommend decongestant nasal spray for involved side. May necessitate immediate referral.
Oroantral fistula (epithelialized oroantral communication	Evaluate radiographs for relationship of roots to the sinus.	Use surgical technique (flaps and tooth/root sectioning) to reduce risk. Do not probe or enlarge socket.	Refer to an oral surgeon for treatment.
TEMPOROMANDIBULAR JOINT			
Trauma	Always acknowledge the potential for TMJ trauma and plan techniques to minimize.	Use bite block or sling support of mandible during extraction. Use **surgical removal** for difficult molar extractions. Shorten time of mouth opening.	Place the patient on a soft diet. Administer heat and analgesics.
Dislocation	Does the patient have a history of previous dislocations?	Same as trauma above.	Manually relocate the joint.
BROKEN INSTRUMENTS			
Elevators	Purchase high-quality elevators.	Use controlled forces. Only use the elevator as it was designed to be used.	Attempt removal; if unsuccessful, refer to an oral and maxillofacial surgeon.
Needles	Purchase disposable needles.	Use only new disposable needles.	Attempt removal; if unsuccessful, refer to an oral and maxillofacial surgeon.

POTENTIAL COMPLICATIONS	PRE-SURGICAL EVALUATION AND PLANNING	PRECAUTIONS DURING SURGERY	MANAGEMENT
BLEEDING	Screen health history for potential bleeding problems. Evaluate anatomy for flap design.	Remove all granulation tissue. Do not tear or crush tissue. Avoid damaging major vessels. Have patient bite on gauze for 15 minutes following surgery before leaving the office.	Apply pressure with gauze. Tie off bleeding vessels. Burnish bone where bleeding. Apply Gelfoam® or Surgicel® to socket.
FIBRINOLYTIC ALVEOLITIS ("Dry Socket")	Inform patient of risk if removing mandibular 3rd molars (the incidence of osteitis following removal of mandibular 3rd molars is greater than 5%).	Use nerve blocks. Carefully debride the wound. Minimize trauma. Apply a broad spectrum antibiotic in the socket (Terra Cortril (Pfizer), tetramycin and cortisone).	Irrigate the socket with warm sterile saline. Place medicated dressing. Repeat daily for 1-2 weeks. Administer strong analgesics for the first few days.
BONE SPICULES		Carefully debride the socket.	Remove with hemostat or curette.
NERVE INJURY	Evaluate radiographs for proximity of tooth to the mandibular canal. Plan flap incisions to avoid mental and lingual nerves.	Use care when sectioning mandibular third molars (may be related to 2nd molar surgery also). Minimize trauma. Use care in reflecting buccal flaps near the mental foramen.	Refer to oral and maxillofacial surgeon experienced in nerve repair.
PAIN	Pre-surgical assessment for elevated pain potential (more emotional patients have more post-op pain).	Minimize trauma. Give initial analgesic dose preoperatively.	Prescribe appropriate analgesics.
SWELLING		Minimize trauma. Place ice packs over area for a few hours post-operatively.	None, unless due to infection. See below.
INFECTION	Avoid elective surgery in areas of non-localized infection (e.g. control moderate to serious cellulitis resulting from pericoronitis prior to surgical extraction of the involved 3rd molar).	Use sterile instruments and aseptic surgical technique. Careful debridement.	See **Diagnosis and Treatment of Odontogenic Infections**, Hohl, et al, Stoma Press, 1983.

REFERENCES

1. Birn, H.: **Etiology and Pathogenesis of Fibrinolytic Alveolitis.** Int J Oral Surg, 2:211-263, 1973.
2. Howe, G.: **Minor Oral Surgery.** Bristol, John Wright and Sons, 1971.
3. Killey, H. C., and Kay, L. W.: **The Prevention of Complications in Dental Surgery.** Eidenburg, Livingston, 1969.
4. Killey, H. C., Seward, G. R., and Kay, L. W.: **An Outline of Oral Surgery.** Bristol, John Wright and Sons, 1971.
5. Kruger: **Textbook of Oral Surgery (Fourth Edition).** The C. V. Mosby Co., St. Louis, 1974.
6. McCarthy: **Emergencies in Dental Practice (Second Edition).** W. B. Saunders Co., Philadelphia, 1972.
7. Schwartz, L. J.: **Lingual Anesthesia Following Mandibular Odontectomy.** J Oral Surg, 31, December 1973.
8. Shira, R.: In McCarthy, F. M.: **Emergencies in Dental Practice.** Philadelphia, Saunders, 1972.
9. Swanson, A. E.: **Reducing the Incidence of Dry Socket: A Clinical Appraisal.** J Can Dent Assoc, 32:25-33, 1966.